WISDOM OF
TAI CHI

ANCIENT SECRETS
TO HEALTH
&
HARMONY

Peter Fenton, Ph.D.
Consultant: Lawrence Galante, Ph.D.

Peter Fenton has a doctorate and a master's degree in educational philosophy and a bachelor's degree in philosophy. His interests cover many fields including natural history, indigenous medical and educational traditions, and world religions. He is the author of numerous articles and technical works including his first book, *Shaolin Nei Jin Qi Gong: Ancient Healing in the Modern World*.

Lawrence Galante holds his doctorate in Health Sciences and an M.A. in Eastern Philosophy and Mysticism. A student of tai chi chuan since 1966, Galante is the president of his own school of tai chi chuan. His extensive training and practice includes tai chi, chi kung, and kung fu. He is certified by the Japanese Shiatsu Association and the Council for Homeopathic Certification. Galante teaches and lectures extensively, and he has written numerous publications including, *Tai Chi: The Supreme Ultimate*, *Tai Chi: Its Form, Function and Application Revealed*, and *Energy Healing: Homeopathy, Chi Kung, Tai Chi and Other Healing Arts*.

TABLE OF CONTENTS

太極

Introduction

This book is intended to be an affirmation of life and joy, of hope and wisdom. It is about the philosophy called Tai Chi, or Great Ultimate, and about tai chi chuan, a martial art whose name means "perfect boxing." Tai chi chuan is much more than a sport or exercise, although this is the way it is popularly understood in the West. It is even more than a martial art. Tai chi chuan is a living philosophy expressed in a series of graceful, complementary, and deeply contemplated movements.

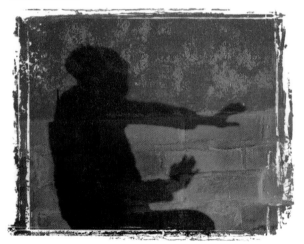

Over the course of centuries, the movements of tai chi chuan have become icons that represent specific ideas—ideas that can be found in ancient philosophical works such as the *I Ching* and the

Tao Te Ching. This book, then, is not devoted exclusively to the martial applications of perfect boxing. Rather, it traces and elucidates the seminal ideas that gave birth to tai chi. We will find these same concepts recurring over vast periods of time in many diverse domains. They figure prominently in myth and legend; in divination practices; in literature, poetry, painting, and calligraphy; in traditional Chinese medicine; in the esoteric arts of Buddhist and Taoist temples; and, of course, in many of the martial arts. Drawing deeply on myth and legend—and the rich metaphors these traditions invoke—*Wisdom of Tai Chi* tells the story of tai chi chuan.

Modern society does not lend itself well to the cultivation of a sophisticated inner life. Nor is it especially conducive to the development of a healthy, robust physical body. Our lives are often hectic, overfilled with distractions and enormous personal responsibilities. This is no secret; we are well aware that our way of life is not only unhealthy but often leads to unhappiness as well.

Radiant health and happiness, however, are our birthright. And tai chi chuan offers us a compelling system that can lead us to reclaiming that birthright. In doing so, we will create an inner sanctuary in which we can develop powerful tools, such as courage and resolve, to utilize in our daily lives. By taking the time and making the effort to learn tai chi chuan, we give ourselves this great gift.

Mythic Origins
of
Taoism

陰陽

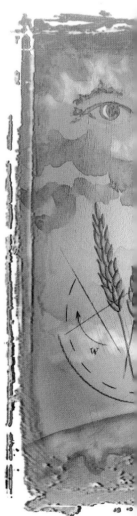

It has been said that mythology is the language of the human soul. A myth speaks to us in ways ordinary language cannot, touching us subtly, almost imperceptibly. Myths speak directly to our hearts. As a result, these stories are empowering. Sometimes they enable us to perceive fundamental truths about our world and those who inhabit it. At other times, they help illuminate people's inner qualities.

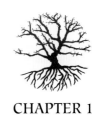

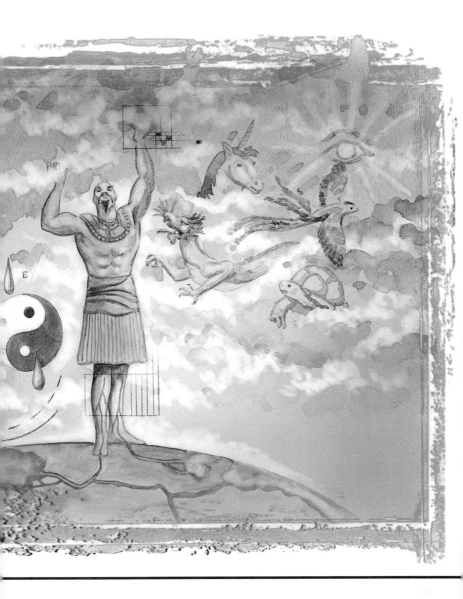

CHAPTER 1

陰陽

The Meaning of Myth

Myths have another special quality. If we read deeply enough into their messages, we find that they sometimes describe our ancestral heritage. As well as telling a simple story, myths often have several layers of meaning. It is not unusual for these deeper layers to be concealed. Like any good secret, this quality provokes our curiosity and leads us gently into reflection on their inner meaning. The great beauty of myths, though, is that these ancient stories speak eloquently for themselves, and their meaning very often unfolds naturally over time.

This happens because myths are vehicles used to recount the common archetypal experiences of our ancestral past. The deep connection with human experience is one reason mythology is universal in its appeal. In this sense, myth is a higher language that enables the wisdom of past generations to survive the ravages of time. Myths endure for two reasons. Firstly, they entertain us. Secondly, they are accessible to all of us, regardless of our age or cultural heritage.

Essentially, though, myths provide a framework that helps us organize our thoughts on difficult matters. While these structures often appear simple enough, their content can be rich in suggestion and hidden meaning. Nowhere is this more apparent than in Chinese mythology. With a tenacity that is sometimes overwhelming, the original ideas expressed by the ancient sages in myths and legends have been preserved, clarified, and organized into entire philosophical systems. The endless discussion, meticulous research, and absolute devotion of several thousand years of Chinese scholarship has ensured their timelessness. As a result, they now lie at the heart of many Chinese disciplines such as poetry, painting, calligraphy, the martial arts, and architecture. They are even the basis of military strategy and board games.

陰陽

The Living Myths of Tai Chi Chuan

In the West, we most often hear myths as stories told through the spoken or written word. But the Chinese have found other ways to pass on the core ideas from their stories and traditions. Tai chi chuan, for example, is a practice that is especially dependent upon the language of movement to transmit its ideas. A particular series of movements, called a form or set, is used to encode and preserve most of the technical infor-

THE ART AND SCIENCE OF TAI CHI

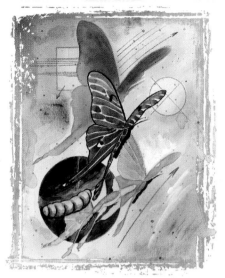

Tai chi chuan is a discipline, providing a structure through which we can express our innermost feelings, beliefs, and ideas. It also offers a means to critique that structure and, when necessary, to change it.

Tai chi chuan is also a tool for examining our roots as human beings and for exploring the potential within us. It begins with a study of the body, for it is through knowing the body that we can understand the mind. Eventually we learn to know ourselves so well that we change. Our metamorphosis is complete. It is one of body, mind, and soul.

In a sense, this transformation can be likened to that of the caterpillar, which incubates in a deathlike trance in the cocoon. One day, along with its skin, it sheds its wormlike form, spreads its wings, and flies off to the nearest flower to drink its nectar.

mation associated with this art. Although to the casual observer a form appears much like a dance, each carries within its framework all of the core philosophy passed on through myth, legend, and the secret traditions of the ages. If students learn the movements of tai chi chuan, they also unavoidably "learn" something about its underlying philosophy.

陰陽

A Taoist Mythology of Creation

When we hear a myth about the creation of the world for the first time, it helps to reflect on a period when our earliest ancestors were searching for answers about things they could not explain. The explanations they came up with, about the soul and about nature, originate in similar kinds of meditations, regardless of the geographical region or historical era. Eventually these ideas were expressed in myths and legends. By studying them, we can reveal the common roots of our humanity.

Long before contemporary scientific and psychological thought, there was aboriginal thought, a mode of thinking that was, and still is, comfortable, even intimate, with myth. Such thinking proceeds from the original, natural mind. It is an outcome of a special, nearly extinct, way of life. In one sense, this type of thinking may be considered unsophisticated and even primitive. In another sense, though, aboriginal thought is a powerful tool. It is a way of deriving conclusions that is simple, direct, and uncluttered by systems of logic and vast vocabularies.

Knowing something about the way of life that gives rise to original thought is important because this knowledge allows us to rediscover facets of ourselves that have been neglected and forgotten.

When the Chinese creation myth is heard for the first time, we see in it a story similar to that told in the Bible, in the Book of Genesis. We also see a tendency in Chinese thought to express concepts in terms of essential components. The primal forces of the masculine and feminine, of the yang and the yin and their permutations, are emphasized. This ability to express abstract ideas in a direct manner is never really abandoned throughout the entire history of Chinese philosophical thought.

Rather than beginning this book with a hefty philosophical account, it is more appropriate to extend an invitation. In a sense, a myth is a kind of invitation. A myth is like a greeting, and it contains a message from the past, offered to the present. Myths introduce us to a particular part, however small, of the prehistory of a civilization.

The Myth of Pan Ku: Creation and the Universal Egg

In the beginning of time, there was only chaos. The elements and gases of the heavens and earth freely mingled, and the organizing principle was dormant. It lay dormant somewhere

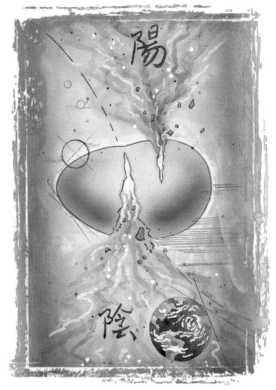

inside this elemental cosmos, awaiting the right moment to begin the transformation. The shape of this primeval mass was something like an egg. For 18,000 years the universe remained in this state, until the incubation was finally complete, and the egg hatched. Then the heavens and the earth came into existence. The lighter, most pure substances floated upward and became the heavens. These elements were named yang. The heavier, more impure substances descended and became the earth. These were named yin.

From the same forces, a third, the giant Pan Ku, was born as well. As he grew, his sheer size divided the heavens and the earth. The giant lived for another 18,000 years. With the assistance of four creatures, a tortoise, a phoenix, a dragon, and a unicorn, he labored daily to mold the earth. Together they created the world as we know it today.

When Pan Ku finally died, his body was transformed. His left eye became the sun and his right eye became the moon. His blood became the rivers and oceans, his breath became the wind, his sweat became the rain, and his voice became the thunder. His flesh became the soil, and from the fleas living on his body, the human race sprang into being. In this way, the stage was set for the pageant of history to unfold.

The story of Pan Ku is the Chinese myth of creation. The ancient myths of creation from virtually all cultures show that at the root of human experience is the belief that our world has an organizing principle. After this creative force appears, everything else takes the form of opposing forces: heaven and earth, black and white, day and night, good and evil. These are the ideas of the yang and the yin, of the masculine and feminine. These opposing qualities are, by their fundamental natures, equal in all respects but forever separate entities. Here we see the theme

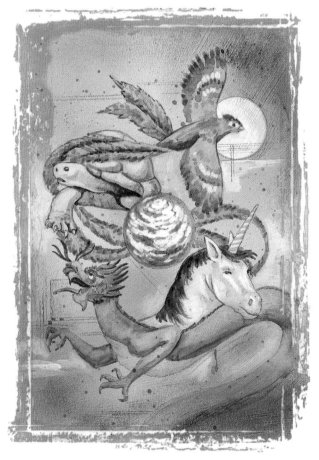

of the One giving rise to the two in the order of creation, and of a creator who, like Pan Ku, works with primordial substances to bring an entire world into being.

陰陽

Nature's Opposing Forces

Simple observation of nature shows us an abundant display of forces in opposition. It is difficult to find more convincing examples of duality than those offered by the natural world. Winter and summer, spring and fall, life and death, hard and soft, high and low tide are all signs that clearly point to the hidden processes of nature. Even if we cannot actually see duality and opposition as fundamental forces, our observations reveal their dramatic consequences. We see that beyond any doubt the yang and the yin, far from being simply abstract concepts, actually represent a dynamic force central to both the animate and inanimate worlds. As the myth of Pan Ku tells us, this universe and everything in it is created, through the grace of the organizing principle, from the interaction of the forces of the yang and the yin.

With deeper study it becomes apparent that, as part of nature, human beings are subject to these basic laws as well. In each of our lives there is a steady rhythmic swing, and we continuously move from one pole to the other. Like a pendulum in its inexorable movement from side to side, the central events in our lives come and go and then return again. Just as certainly as the tide rises and falls, the vigor of youth will turn to the weakness of age. We also know that all things

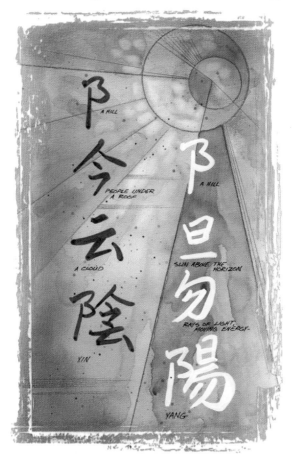

pass; in time, sorrow fades, making room for joy. Ignorance, with effort and persistence, can be transformed into wisdom. The forces at play in the world take from the one side and give to the other. As we observe the endless ebb and flow of the tides, the constant cycle of day and night, and the movement through life from youth to old age, life displays for us the world and all of its interactions in terms of these relationships.

Understanding this basic concept, we can search out clues to help us to make accurate judgments about ourselves and others, about relationships, and about possibilities and limitations. The sign of health and prosperity, for example, is a well-balanced life. In a similar way, the sign of wisdom is the ability to balance both the pleasures and demands of life. There is a wise saying, "you cannot take blood from a stone," which suggests that before every attempt, it would be advantageous to consider the inherent limitations of every act as well as its possibilities.

Tai Chi: Symbol of The Great Ultimate

This theme of opposing forces became particularly important in Taoist thought, where it is represented in symbolic form. The illustration on the facing page depicts the creation myth just described. Pan Ku is shown holding an egg-shaped shield representing the universe before creation. Engraved on the shield is a symbol often used in Taoism. It is that of the Tai Chi, The Great Ultimate, which represents the primal, creative forces of yin and yang in a state of perfect balance. The forces are represented by the black (yin) and the white (yang) halves. But the line that separates the two halves is not straight.

Instead, it is curved, symbolizing the potential for dynamic interaction between the polarized forces. In the center of each half is a small, empty circle. In the dark half, the circle is light, and in the light half, it is dark. These small dots denote

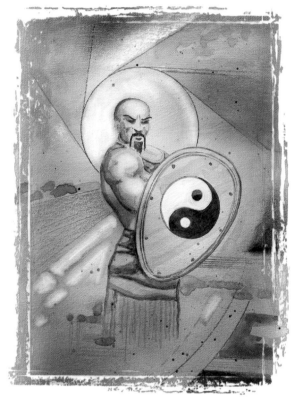

the seeds of change impregnating the wombs. Mastering these forces, the giant is able to create the world and everything in it. Symbolically, Pan Ku represents the giant in each of us who is capable of mastering the powerful, natural forces of which we are made.

陰陽
Symbols in Language and Culture

The most important myths have, over time, all been transformed into icons. These icons are symbols that tell stories without words. As such, they may contain many layers of meaning. Most of the time, the symbols and their deeper meanings remain hidden from our conscious mind. We may unconsciously understand the veiled meanings of the symbols, or we may not. In either case, they most certainly exert a powerful influence on us.

Imagine, for example, a group of people entering a very large cathedral. First they see the windows, stained glass that has darkened with age, depicting dramatic biblical scenes. There may be statues here and there and other religious artifacts. Even the architecture of the cathedral itself has been designed to evoke a religious feeling. Whether or not individuals in the group are conscious of this, the effect will be the same. Upon entering the cathedral, they will likely all fall silent. Some will become emotional. Everyone will experience a change in mood. Such is the power of symbol.

Symbols and their Messages

What makes a symbol powerful is the body of knowledge behind it. Taken out of context, a symbol is essentially without meaning. This can

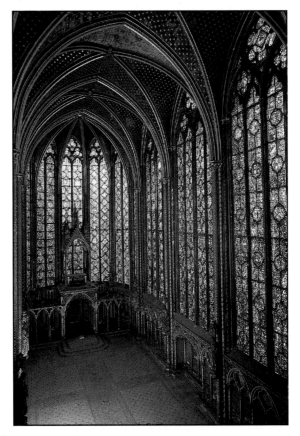

be seen even today in our modern world. Each year, patent offices worldwide process countless requests to patent particular symbols. Once society recognizes a symbol, it becomes a powerful tool in the world of marketing and advertising.

Graphic artists are highly paid to conceive of symbols that will resonate with people and gain the attention of the buying public. This only happens because that symbol brings to mind the whole idea of the product—what it can do for us, how it tastes, or why we need it. Around this symbol, a product or line of products is marketed.

In the past, though, symbols were created for another reason. They were used as a means of encoding information in a way that could be conveniently remembered and recorded. In fact, this is exactly how both spoken and written language developed. Words represent objects as well as ideas. At first words were only spoken. Later, pictorial images were used to represent these words. In some cases, such as the English language, the images have become so abstracted from their original meaning that it is no longer possible to see the relationship. This is not true of the Chinese language. Its symbols can still be traced to original meanings.

The Chinese have proven themselves adept at creating highly abstract systems of symbols that encompass large bodies of knowledge. History also attests to their remarkable ability to integrate new symbols and new ideas into an existing system of thought. The Chinese system of traditional medicine, for example, is based not only on concepts and techniques arising from within their own culture, but also on ideas from many foreign lands, including India and Tibet.

The long-term effect of this tendency is the formation of a worldview that is comprehensive, systematic, and rigorous. This progressive development is apparent in many Chinese disciplines including acupuncture, herbal lore, philosophy, literature, painting, calligraphy, and the martial arts. Many of the fundamental ideas supporting this worldview are described in the book known as the *I Ching*.

陰陽

The *I Ching*

A very early system of symbols is found in the *I Ching*, considered to be an ancient text even among the Chinese themselves, who boast a very long recorded history. Among other things, the *"I,"* as it is known, is a treatise on the practice of divination, or foretelling the future. When discussing Chinese philosophy it is difficult to avoid turning to the *I Ching*. In the same way that mythology sparks both the imagination and the intellect, so, too, does the *"I."*

For this reason, it is one of the most consulted and commented on books ever written. To those who understand it, it is certainly one of the most cherished. Although it presents the concept of an orderly, structured universe, the writings are puzzling because of their extensive reliance on very old images and metaphors. This quality not only indicates its considerable age, but is, perhaps, the source of its greatness, since these writings demand that its readers use both intuition and open-minded thinking. The writings require us to reflect on the meaning of a very basic and ancient set of ideas.

In the context of the book itself, the Chinese word "I" refers to "change." For this reason, the text is known in the English language as *The Book of Changes*. The word "I" also refers to the notions of "simplicity" and "ease." This suggests a deep connection with the natural world. What could be easier or more simple than a life guided by instinct?

Even though scholars believe this book to be one of the oldest in existence, it is used even today as both a tool to investigate the permutations of life and as an oracle. Research in this century has arrived at a number of conclusions about the *I Ching*'s history, about its uses in the past, and also about its meaning. One of the most interesting features of the book is that its creation has been something of a community effort. With the passage of centuries, devotees have added extensive commentary. The most famous of all commentators was the sage Confucius, whose writings, together with those of his contemporary Lao Tsu, formed the backbone of subsequent Chinese philosophical thought. Confucius is believed to have added at least some of the commentaries known as the *Ten Wings*. These masterworks were written as supplements to the older parts of the book. The older chapters, consolidated with the newer commentaries, form a single, cohesive work that is the basis of *The Book of Changes* we read today.

The *I Ching* and Its Symbols

We have seen how the shape of Pan Ku's shield represents the cosmic egg and how the

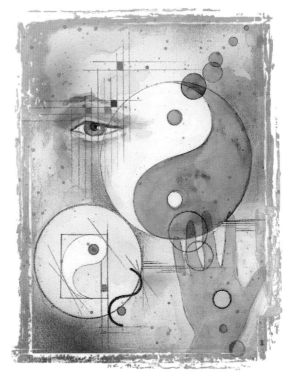

interplay of the two cosmic forces, the yin and the yang, are represented by the black and the white halves of the Tai Chi symbol. But there are still

THE EIGHT FORCES OF NATURE AND THEIR TRIGRAMS

The following table describes the relationship between each trigram and its corresponding natural force. Heaven is represented as three solid lines and expresses a masculine, aggressive, and creative force. Within this system of lines and broken lines, it is visually clear how the three solid lines form a ladder heavenward, leading to the abode of the gods. Earth, the polar opposite of heaven, is represented by three broken lines, and represents receptivity and fertility. These are classified into the eight houses shown in the table below.

When two separate trigrams are coupled, a hexagram or six-lined figure results. By coupling the original eight trigrams in all possible configurations, 64 combinations result. Together these are used to symbolize the major categories of human experience.

⚊ ⚊ ⚊	⚋ ⚋ ⚋	⚋ ⚋ ⚊	⚋ ⚊ ⚋	⚊ ⚋ ⚋	⚊ ⚊ ⚋	⚊ ⚋ ⚊	⚋ ⚊ ⚊
Heaven: *House of the Creative*	**Earth:** *House of the Receptive*	**Thunder:** *House of the Arousing*	**Water:** *House of the Abysmal*	**Mountain:** *House of the Keeping Still*	**Wind:** *House of the Gentle*	**Fire:** *House of the Clinging*	**Lake:** *House of the Joyous*

The Eight Primal Forces and the Corresponding Trigrams

deeper levels of meaning. The small dots, or seeds of change, which inhabit the yang and the yin portions of the Tai Chi, symbolize the dynamics of growth, development, and change. These are the ideas which preceded and encouraged the first attempts at prediction and divination.

陰陽

Divination and Knowledge

It is very likely that before the *I Ching*, sets of bones were cast in an attempt to know the future. These oracle bones, unearthed by archaeologists, were precursors to the divination system that is now used in the *"I,"* either a set of 50 yarrow sticks or a set of three coins.

Essentially, the *I Ching* is a system that has always been used to predict the future. More importantly, though, is its use as a book of wisdom. Because the readings it gives are simple, yet elegant, profound, and intuitive, it is often consulted for its advice and insight into human nature. It is also read simply as an account of human affairs. In many circles, the book is no less influential today than it was hundreds of years ago.

Just like the Judeo-Christian Bible, there is no certainty as to who actually wrote much of the

THE FLOWERING OF YIN
AND YANG

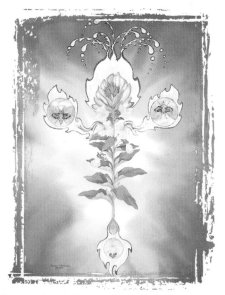

The evening primrose is an excellent example of
the balance of yin and yang. This plant circulates
energy beautifully. Its tall, symmetrical stature gives
us a clue to its special ability to achieve a perfect equi-
librium between these two dynamic forces. With its
fire energy, it carries the life force heavenward along
its central axis, the stem, and emanates that energy
outward through its leaves and brilliant yellow blossoms as it proceeds on its ascension.

The yin energy of the evening primrose is exem-
plified in its relationship to the sphinx moth. It is the
host plant for this moth, which is almost as big as a
hummingbird. Without the nurturing and receptivity
of the primrose's fragrant blossoms, the moth could
not be sustained.

I Ching. Sometime close to the dawn of recorded history, the main text itself came into being. About 3,000 years ago, during the Zhou dynasty, the first records of its existence appear.

Even then, the philosophers of the time recognized the fundamental principles already touched upon—that in the beginning exists Tai Chi, The Great Ultimate, and from it springs the yin and the yang. The yin is symbolized in *The Book of Changes* by a broken line (- -) and the yang, by a solid line (–). How better to indicate a yielding, nurturing force than with a broken line and an active, aggressive force with a solid line?

Yin, Yang, and the Forces of Change

As has been suggested, yin is regarded as the feminine principle—nurturing, reflective, and yielding in character. Yang is considered the masculine force—active, intellectual, and dominant. Although they are opposites, the two forces complement each other. In their permutations and interactions, they are the forces responsible for the constant change we see in the world.

In terms of making predictions about the future, we can use our knowledge of yang and yin to come to some conclusions. We know, for example, that everything in this world is subject to change. Day will give way to night in the same way that summer will yield to winter. At the same time, we can see patterns and cycles within this framework of change. These patterns, for exam-

UNIVERSAL PRINCIPLES

In the modern world, the idea of divination is often ridiculed. How could it be possible, the argument goes, to predict the future by interpreting the turn of a card or the toss of some coins? But the system of hexagrams represents a very significant development in philosophical thought. It interprets both the visible and invisible worlds as being subject to universal laws. Since all worlds must operate according to a formal set of principles, as long as our tools are adequate and our interpretations accurate, we can gain insight into the future. Such a system was, and is, absolutely impartial. Even the gods, in spite of their magical abilities, are governed by these laws.

The ancient Greeks and many other cultures from antiquity did not, at first, have any such system. To disclose the future, they had to rely on an intermediary, such as the Delphic Oracle, to petition a particular god. The oracle would then explain the feelings of the god, who was by no means bound to act in accordance with fundamental principles. If the god was feeling slighted, offended, jealous, angry, irritable, or playful, it was likely there would be a terrible scene in which unfortunate mortals invariably suffered.

So, in this scheme of things, the vision of the future was not dependent upon the interplay of impartial natural forces, but on the whims of all-powerful deities. The mechanisms of the I Ching, on the other hand, suggest a world guided by the superior influences of universal principles rather than governed by the whims of an emotional god.

ple, often repeat themselves with mathematical precision. We have also determined that the patterns, such as the 24-hour cycle of a day or the 12-month cycle of a year, will exhibit extremes of both yang and yin at different times. Knowing this, we can easily make simple projections about the future. Events such as the moment of sunrise or the exact time and date of a high tide can now be predicted with relative ease. It was not always so. The first mathematicians who learned through their science to predict such events as a solar eclipse were regarded as wizards, and it is surprising that more of them were not executed as a result. These types of predictions, though, dealt largely with what we in the West consider to be the inanimate world.

By investigating more closely still, we can see that living things, including ourselves, are also subject to these same processes. Since these processes do not change and are always governing how we behave, they are considered to be universal laws. Once this idea is accepted, it is not so difficult to see how a system of divination with specifically human applications might be constructed.

The *I Ching* System

First, this system needs to organize the general categories of human experience. Then it must devise a method of evaluating which of these events would be most likely to happen at a particular time for a particular person. To their eternal credit, the authors of the *I Ching* have constructed just such a system.

By using the solid line (–) to represent yang and the broken line (- -) to represent yin, the *I Ching* can symbolically express a relationship between the two forces. The only drawback is that by using just these two symbols, only four relationships can be expressed, the relation of yang to itself (two solid lines), the relation of yin to itself (two sets of broken lines) and their relation to each other (two more cases with either a yin line on the bottom or a yang line on the bottom). The genius of the *I Ching* is that to create more categories, it organizes the two forces of yin and yang into sets of three separate lines, called the trigram. Now there are eight possibilities. Finally, each separate trigram is coupled with another trigram. From these two groups of three lines, one larger group of six lines is created. This is referred to as a hexagram.

The Trigrams and the Eight Forces of Nature

When grouped into threes, yin and yang now have eight possible combinations. In their wisdom, the ancient sages used these categories to symbolize the eight primeval forces of nature. When grouped into sixes, yin and yang have 64 possible combinations. The sages used these to describe the life situations common to all humanity.

THE TREE OF BIFURCATION

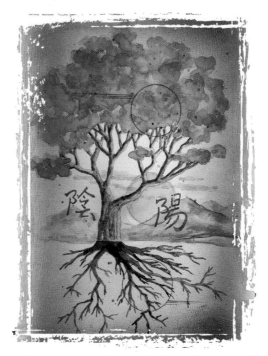

This artistic rendering of what is known as "The Tree of Bifurcation" illustrates the progressive development of the 64 hexagrams. In the beginning there was the One, represented by the roots of a tree. Just above the ground, the root branches into two forks. Convention has it that the left fork represents the yin and the right, the yang. Each fork branches again, making four branches, and again making eight. These eight branches, of course, are the eight primal forces: Earth, mountain, water, and wind are yin; thunder, fire, lake, and heaven are yang. Two more sets of branches make 16 and 32; a final branch completes the set at 64, all of which are named in the I Ching.

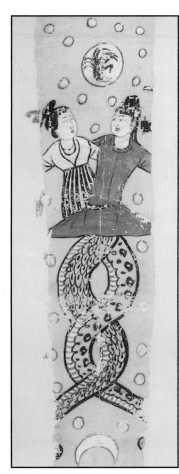

The origins of the eight trigrams are traditionally ascribed to the mythic ruler Fu-Hsi (Fuxi), who, as a divine being, had the body of a snake. According to the story, Fu-Hsi gave several incomparable gifts to humanity, including the skills of animal husbandry and fishing with nets. He also created musical instruments and a system of writing using knotted cords. Most importantly for the purpose at hand, he is credited with the development of the system of the eight trigrams.

His purpose in developing the trigrams was to organize all phenomena under heaven and earth and to place them within a simple and comprehensive framework. When arranged in a circular pattern around the Tai Chi symbol, the

notation became known as Pa-Kua, the philosophical precursor of the *I Ching*. The symbols of
Pa-Kua were likely devised as abstractions of the
ancient myths. Given their original purpose, it is
no wonder that the trigrams became the basis for
the practice of divination.

One of the most appealing features about this
system is its simplicity. According to its theory, all
phenomena can be grouped according to one of
eight principle trigrams, each of which becomes an
icon in the process. The symbol identified as
Heaven, for example, also encompasses such concepts as ruler, wealth, day, and father, to name just
a few. Several thousand years ago, the world was
very unlike our own. The world was then, it seems,
much more straightforward and less complex. As
the world changed, so did the system of Pa-Kua
until it eventually developed into the comprehensive system of analysis known as the *I Ching*.

The Hexagrams

Not until the 12th century did the relatively
complex system of 64 hexagrams come into
being. The ruler Wen Wang, of the Hsi-Chou
Dynasty, developed Pa-Kua until it became the
sophisticated analytical tool we know today. As
we have seen, the hexagram is formed by six
lines, either broken or solid. Surprising as it may
seem, the rationale for using six lines for a successful divination, and not some other number, is
still with us. In each of the lower and upper tri-

EIGHT PRIMAL FORCES AND TRADITIONAL CHINESE MEDICINE

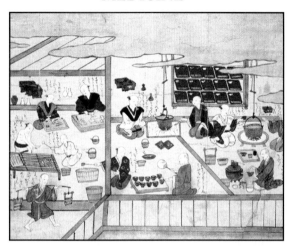

Traditional Chinese medical diagnosis adopted a type of description inspired by the primal forces of nature. Even today, patients are diagnosed as having too much fire or too much cold. When out of balance, the raw forces of nature have unfortunate consequences for the patient. The wise physician perceives imbalances by studying physiological clues. The physician may discover these imbalances during a discussion with the patient (known as the interrogation) or by examining the urine, tongue, complexion, pulse, and other physiological indicators. After the investigation, the physician may prescribe herbal preparations, a change in lifestyle, a different diet, a new outlook on life or, most likely, some combination of these remedies. The sole purpose of the prescription is to bring the energies in the body back into balance.

grams, one line is assigned to heaven, one to the earth, and one to humanity. The six lines are arranged in a stack that is separated into two parts, an upper half and a lower half. This stack forms the basis of the predictive readings given in the *I Ching*. The basic part of this text is simply

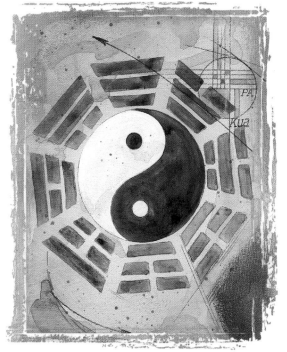

The Pa-Kua

64 explanations, one for each of the hexagrams. When a hexagram is cast, the *I Ching* is then consulted for insight into its meaning.

Each of the six lines is assigned a special meaning according to its relative position to the others in the stack. A broken line on the bottom

DIGITALIS: NATURE'S OWN
DANCE OF WATER AND FIRE

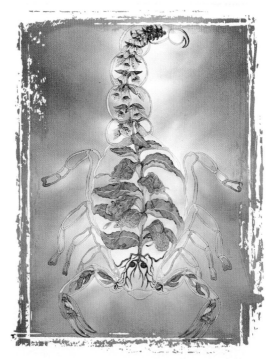

*The elements of water and fire are perfectly bal-
anced in the foxglove plant* (digitalis purpurea). *Foxglove's fire energy is its deadly poison, which can stop
the heart instantly. When used with medical precision,
however, the same poison keeps the heart beating.*

*The foxglove plant also has a serene character,
the influence of the water element, the plant's governing force. Nature never makes a mistake. She has created balance, taking two conflictive forces to make
something of beauty and power. This is the kind of
transformation the* I Ching *seeks to help us with in
our own affairs.*

of the stack, for example, might indicate some kind of fundamental weakness, whereas a solid line might suggest the opposite. So the *I Ching* explains the meaning of the hexagram as a whole and also discusses each of the six lines as separate entities. This in-depth analysis makes for a simple but logical system.

Each hexagram within the framework is of equal value. They are all neutral. They cannot be described as being either good or bad in themselves, but they do contain the seeds of either favorable or unfavorable possibilities. It is here that the commentaries in the *Ten Wings* reveal a wonderful secret. The commentaries show us that each of the hexagrams can be interpreted in two ways, known as the superior and the inferior outlooks. With a superior outlook, the reading will offer clues as to how best to deal with forthcoming situations.

It would be a simple matter to slip into the mistake of believing that one divination was superior to another. In a tarot card reading, for example, it is easy to think that drawing the Death card is a portent of misfortune. After all, the Death card often bears the illustration of a skeleton. But what is important in a hexagram reading, like the Tarot, is not the superficial appearance of the card, or the toss of the coins, but the information that the selection conveys, the interpretation that is rendered, and how the ideas can be applied in life.

So, as explained earlier, all hexagrams are inherently neutral. They indicate conditions in both the inner and outer worlds as they surround the diviner. If these indications are indeed correct, it is theoretically possible to prepare for events, regardless of what they might be, in an appropriate manner. In this way disaster may avoided, and favorable circumstances can be exploited to the maximum.

Casting the Hexagram

In the past, 50 yarrow sticks were used to perform an *I Ching* divination. These were selected from plants with tall, straight stalks. At that time, plants were believed to have a direct contact with the source of creation. The yarrow *(Achillea millefolium)*, known also as milfoil or tansy, is well-known throughout the world. In ancient China, it was held in high regard as a particularly sacred plant. Its prominence may be the result of its special curative power—it promotes blood clotting.

Since this method of divination is difficult to use, a modern method was devised that uses a set of three coins. In this system, the head of the coin represents yang and has a value of three. Tails represents yin and has a value of two. The three coins are tossed, and one of four possible combinations will result. When added together, the numbers on all three coins will total either six, seven, eight, or nine.

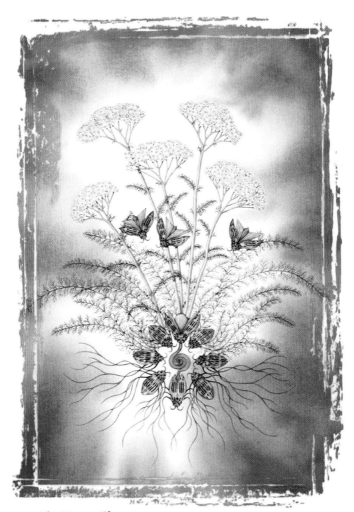

The Yarrow Plant

To cast a hexagram, toss three coins and add the values. Draw the first line according to the chart on the next page and place it at the bottom of the stack. Throw the coins five more times, making six lines in all. This is a hexagram.

Coin Cast Associations

Coin Cast	Numerical Value	Polarity	Line Type
3 heads	9	yang	moving
3 tails	6	yin	moving
2 heads, 1 tail	8	yin	broken
2 tails, 1 head	7	yang	solid

The system is further enhanced by adding the idea of "old" lines and "young" lines. An old line can be either yin or yang depending on its proximity to its opposite. We have discussed the idea of the eternal movement of energy and the constant change that this movement brings. Like an ocean tide at its height, an old yang line has reached its peak and is at the point of retreat. Soon it will begin its transformation back into yin. These special types of lines are referred to as "moving" because they are at the point of change.

A moving line is created when either three heads or three tails are thrown. A toss of three heads would yield a number value of nine. Three tails yield a value of six. Moving lines, after they are changed to their opposite, form a second hexagram that leads to an additional reading that is used in conjunction with the original divination. A hexagram with moving lines, and its derivative, would look like this:

Original Hexagram   Derived Hexagram

6	– –		—
9	—		– –
7	—		—
7	—		—
6	– –		—
7	—		—

The extra hexagram adds an entirely new dimension to the reading. With the original cast of the coins, there were 64 possible combinations. But if a second hexagram derives from the first, then there are 4,096 (64×64) possible combinations. Not every hexagram that is cast will contain a moving line. If it does, however, there is additional information to consider in the analysis.

A Reading from the Text

Here is an interpretation of the hexagram cast above. The reading is a compilation of ideas taken from a number of texts including *The I Ching* or *Book of Changes* by Richard Wilhelm and *I Ching* by Kerson and Rosemary Huang.

The hexagram described above is number 49, meaning Ko or Revolution. Since it happens to be a hexagram with two moving lines, there is a derivative hexagram, number 37, to consider as well. By comparing the hexagram to the table of the eight primal forces (page 26), we find that in the original hexagram, the upper trigram refers to lake and the lower to fire. So, in its most elementary form, the meaning is simply, Lake over Fire.

This hexagram is one of the eight that falls under the House of the Abysmal. Fire consumes and rises. Water extinguishes and falls. The interpretation notes that when water is found above fire, there may be conflict: The fire is extinguished by the fall of the water, and the water, in its turn, evaporates as the fire rises to consume it.

To the ancients, water over fire indicated Revolution, which is the title of the hexagram. The reading, or judgment, as it is called, is an interpretation of the specific meanings of each of the lines. Each line can be difficult to interpret since its original meaning was conceived of hundreds of years ago. As a result, the symbolism is often obscure. The first line, for example, located in the first place at the bottom of the hexagram, is made by three heads and so has a value of nine. At this particular location, nine means something like, "tied with the hide of a yellow ox."

This translates as follows: The hide is tough, strong, and resilient, and therefore suggests determination. As a color, yellow is traditionally associated with forces in balance. As an omen, the hint is to not act prematurely and to wait for an appropriate moment. The ox, or cow, signifies submission, and this confirms the meaning of the earlier clues. Submit, at least temporarily, but remain firm in your convictions.

In terms of a revolution, then, or some planned action against the existing state of affairs, the general message is one of remaining firm and of biding one's time until conditions are more favorable. The entire reading supports this theme. It says: "Justice will be handed down publicly so that all will be aware of the fate of transgressors. This is auspicious for those who have behaved with loyalty and virtue."

陰陽

Intuition and Interpretation

At the core of the I Ching is a method of interpretation that relies on intuition. While suggestions from the text are offered, the final meaning must be determined by those who cast the coins. This is only possible through deep reflection about our personal situation in life. Through the suggestions found in the I Ching, we have a tool to investigate areas in our lives that might otherwise be overlooked. Once we come face to face with these recommendations, it is much more difficult to deny, ignore, misidentify, or misunderstand situations that may require our attention.

We can depend on the *I Ching* to be thorough. Remember that its 64 hexagrams are grouped under eight houses, which themselves represent the eight primal forces of nature. As far as we are concerned, the houses represent the eight principle conditions of life. By virtue of our humanity, all of us are subject to the laws that govern those houses. The hexagram we cast explains these laws to us in detail, so that we are encouraged to attend to the relevant matters in our lives. Whether or not there is any working relationship between the coins we toss to derive a hexagram and our actual life situation is not of paramount importance. What does matter is that we use the cues offered by the *I Ching* to study our own lives. The text would be valuable even if we studied hexagram readings randomly.

If this text can be said to have a heart, then this simple idea must be it. Because of its simplicity and directness, the information presented in the book has great power. It has an uncanny ability to put us in touch with the deeper layers of our minds and the vast storehouse of knowledge each of us possesses unconsciously.

Unless one has profound intuitive abilities, access to these levels is usually only possible through dream analysis, hypnosis, or in certain situations, by therapeutic analysis. Fortunately, the *I Ching* still exists. As a result, we have a simple, gentler method to probe the hidden regions of our minds. To use this system, one must understand the system of divination and recognize that the *I Ching* is a means to communicate with our innermost selves, not just an attempt at prediction or a commentary on life's possibilities.

Centuries of research now accompany the original text. Of course, the additional commentaries are often very valuable and offer great insights into the meaning of the primary work. But they also have the dubious effect of obscuring the original intention. The purpose of the text is to put each of us in touch with the source of our own creativity and inspiration, not to lead us by the hand toward the visions of others.

Ideally, *The Book of Changes* is read with a fresh and open mind, leaving room for its archetypal images to work their own magic. Later, after we become well-versed in the *I Ching* and have formed our own conclusions, the commentaries offer great insight. This strategy allows the ideas of others to assume a place of secondary importance, as the original authors intended. *The Book of Changes* becomes a tool of great personal significance. For those who practice faithfully with the *I Ching*, this is exactly what happens.

Taoism:
A Philosopy and a Way of Life

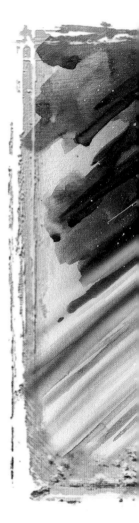

Every language, culture, and religion has words that convey more than one simple idea. Even though such words often have several layers of meaning, there is never any confusion as to what is being said. Ask a dozen people, for example, to explain the word "heaven"—as likely as not, you'll hear a dozen different definitions or descriptions. The same is true of the Chinese word "Tao," which is often translated as "way" or "path."

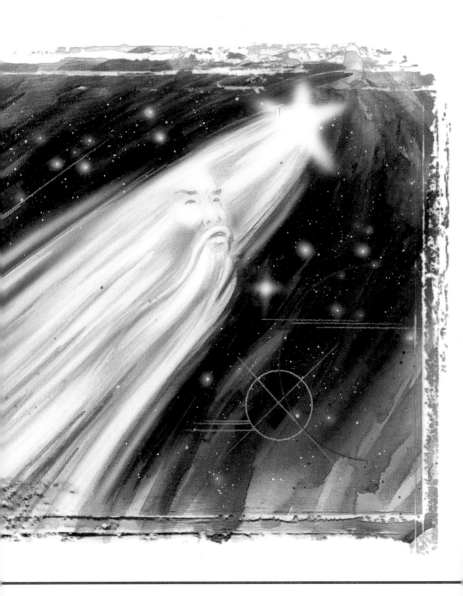

CHAPTER 2

道
The Tao

Although there are many definitions of Tao, this one word communicates an entire philosophy, an outlook on the fundamental nature of life and the universe. The word Tao is nothing less than an expression of the profound unity of the universe and of the path human beings must take to join, rather than disturb, that unity.

What is this path, and how do we find it? The path begins with an understanding of the origin of the universe. "Knowing the ancient beginning is the essence of the way," stated the ancient Chinese sage Lao Tzu, the author of the *Tao Te Ching*. Known in English as *The Book of the Way,* this poetic masterpiece was written approximately 2,500 years ago. As well as being a matchless work of literature, it takes its place in history as the first written record of Taoist philosophy.

The Story of Creation

The Taoist theory of creation is not unlike other traditional creation stories. At first, there was simply a great void, the ultimate quiescence, called "Wu Chi." Wu Chi is also understood as creative potential, primal force, and universal energy. Wu Chi, the source, created the two opposites: yang, the active force, and yin, the passive force. These two forces are perpetually

THE BIRTH OF LAO TZU AND
THE *TAO TE CHING*

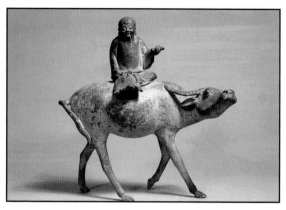

According to legend, Lao Tzu was conceived immaculately in the womb of a shooting star. He was born more than six decades later with a full white beard. His name means "Old Child."

Lao Tzu was a record keeper of the Imperial archives in the ancient capital city of Loyang. One day, distressed with the lifestyle of his contemporaries and their refusal to adopt The Way, he rode away on a water buffalo. Arriving at the great wall that enclosed the civilized world, he was stopped by a sentinel, who had dreamed of the great sage's approach.

The watchman convinced the old philosopher to outline his ideas before leaving. So it was that the Tao Te Ching came into being. After completing this task, Lao Tzu and his buffalo rode off into the vast surrounding desert and were never heard from again. Lao Tzu seems to have left this world as mysteriously as he entered it. In perfect harmony with his teachings, he eventually abandoned what he could not change.

changing, one into the other; their interplay gives birth to the transformation of matter, called "the 10,000 things"—the Taoist expression for everything in the universe. When the perfect balance between yin and yang is achieved, there is harmony, epitomized by the Tai Chi (yin-yang) symbol. Tao is found first by encompassing, and then by balancing, the extremes of both polarities.

Lao Tzu's *Tao Te Ching*, an extraordinary work of 81 mysterious and beautiful verses, offers council for wounded hearts, a path for the lost, and a balm for troubled brows. This compendium of Taoist thought begins:

> The Tao that can be told
>   is not the true Tao.
> The name that can be named
>   is not the eternal name.
> The nameless is the beginning
>   of heaven and earth.
> The named is the mother
>   of the ten thousand things.
> Ever desireless,
>   one can see the mystery.
> Ever desiring, one can see
>   the manifestations.
> These two spring from the same
>   source but differ in name;
>   this appears as darkness.
> Darkness within darkness.
> The gate to all mystery.

Enigmatic and mystical, like all Taoist poetry, this first verse unveils the Taoist understanding of creation and the mystical path of the Tao. It tells us that about Wu Chi, the ultimate void, the eternal, we can say nothing. Its depths are beyond our reaches. We can only reflect on its manifestations: the yin and yang and all that these two forces create; that is, the world we live in and all that is in it. But the study of the interplay between these two forces is enough to start us on the path. By seeking harmony within ourselves, and between ourselves and the outside world and all its inhabitants, we will be able to achieve a superior state of being. By existing in this state of perpetual balance, we develop a true perspective on the nature of life and its unseen source.

Whoever achieves this state achieves "teh," often translated as virtue in the sense of perfection. The person who does not seek to live in harmony with the Tao will remain lopsided with desire, never being able to see things as they are and never comprehending more than what the physical world offers. Lao Tzu makes it clear from the outset that when we search for Tao, we do so without the tools of intellect and language. Using these tools would put the Tao forever beyond our grasp. So it is on the strength of our natural intuitions, guided by the images of poets and painters, that we walk the path, speechlessly seeking Tao, the inexpressible.

道
The Interdependence of All Things

The early Taoist philosophers were profoundly influenced by their observations of nature. They determined that everything has its complementary opposite. More than this, they saw that everything can only be understood by comparing it to its opposite. Day is only day in relation to night, cold only cold in relation to heat, and soft only soft in relation to hard. Looking deeper still, they realized that these relationships are in a constant state of flux: Day flows gradually into night and back again. All things, then, are interdependent. By observing the processes of nature, the Taoists say, we can come to some understanding about the meaning of our lives and about our place in the world. These concepts are the cornerstone of Taoist thought.

Taoist philosophers also noticed that what happens in nature is effortless. This does not mean that there is no struggle, but that events occur without premeditation. Consider the life of a plant. The seed falls onto the ground. If the soil is fertile, and if it receives warmth, light, and water, it may emerge as a seedling. It does not require instruction to know how to take nourishment in through its roots or how to photosynthesize light and unfold into a mature plant.

Given the knowledge it contains, the plant is complete within its own nature. Why should life be

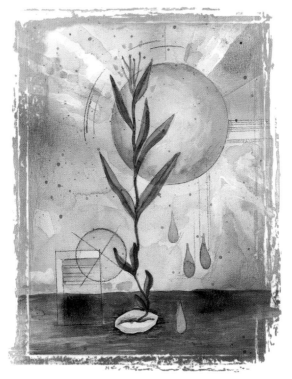

different for people, the Taoist asks? Why not allow situations to unfold as they may rather than trying to manipulate others and orchestrate events. This belief is known as the doctrine of doing-by-not-doing, and it lies at the heart of Taoist practice. It is the message of the following portion of Verse 29 of the *Tao Te Ching:* *(continued on page 58)*

THE DANDELION—AN EXUBERANT TAOIST

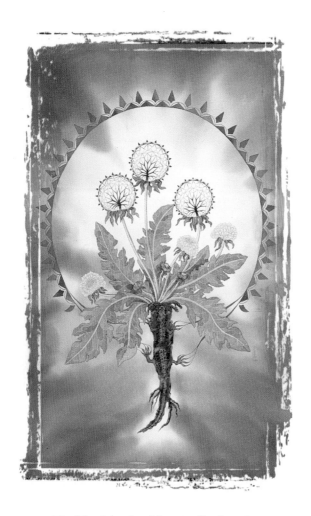

*The life of the dandelion is effortless. It com-
munes perfectly with all the forces of nature so
that it may live out its cycle. In order to disperse*

its seed, the dandelion is equipped with a most beautiful umbrella that breaks apart in the wind. The seeds are carried through air, land softly on the ground, and then take root in the earth. After they are nurtured by the warmth of the sun, by the rain, and by the rich soil, each seed sends a long root deep into the earth. There it begins to make use of the minerals it finds. From the root grow vitamin-rich leaves and yellow blossoms. Then these blossoms use the power of the sun to mature and once again become the seed heads that carry the life force to other destinations. Not only is the dandelion self-perpetuating, its ingenious processes enable it to thrive wherever it finds itself.

Many of us think of the dandelion as a frustrating weed. It invades our manicured lawns and gardens, displacing the grass and flowers we have so carefully planted there. But that is just our misunderstanding of nature, wishing we could control it as we try to control everything else that is natural. Because it is capable of transforming the elements, the dandelion has great potential for humankind. Its leaves are a rich source of vitamins, particularly vitamins A, B_2, and C, and of the mineral calcium, should we decide to use them as a food source. Its root makes a delicious hot drink, and its medicinal uses are many. The root has diuretic properties that may help lower blood pressure, and it has been used to treat liver diseases such as jaundice and cirrhosis. Most of all, the dandelion serves as a living example of the Tao.

Do you think you can take
  over the universe
  and improve it?
I do not believe it can be done.
The universe is sacred.
You cannot improve it.
If you try to change it,
  you will ruin it.
If you try to hold it,
  you will lose it.

Nature is complete without us, this verse tells us. We must recognize this fact and begin to participate with nature as a partner in the universal scheme. Our mission, say the Taoist philosophers, is to return to a natural way of life, unencumbered by complicated social institutions and intellectual ideas. Doing so, they suggest, will return us to a state of natural grace—Tao. This contact with what is innately pure will, in turn, strengthen our spirit, the source of which is nature.

道
Finding The Way

Finding Tao seems impossible at first. In order to understand it, we are told, we must rely on our spirit, not our intellect. Yet we are conditioned to understand things in three ways:

through our instincts and emotions, through our senses, and through the logic of our intellects. Instincts and emotions tell us how we feel about different situations. Our five senses show us what is happening in the world around us. Finally, we draw conclusions with our minds. Each of these ways of knowing represents a different type of understanding. Together they form the boundaries of ordinary experience. The paradox is that knowing through Tao lies beyond these conventional methods. Only by cultivating our spirit, we are told, can we rise above everyday experience.

The Chinese term *shen* means something like the English word "spirit." The meanings, however, are not exactly the same. Shen is thought of as a physical substance, as real as blood or bones. Like everything else to the Chinese, shen is either in or out of balance. When it is balanced and exists in the body in a proper measure, it is said to be developed.

Developing the spirit is possible by relying on two aspects of our mind, referred to as the emotional mind, or *hsin*, and the wisdom mind, or *yi*. Hsin can be used to awaken shen, but yi must be used to control it. If this control is not exerted, problems such as sleeplessness and mental disorder develop. When the control is found, however, great feats can be accomplished. For this reason, Taoists and Buddhists both practice methods especially designed to sublimate emotional energy.

Cultivating spirit, then, requires mastery of both the emotional and intellectual realms of understanding. To control spirit, we must use our minds to control the raw powers of emotion that activate it. Finally, we must express shen through the deeds of our physical bodies. By doing so, we will effortlessly display a balance that reflects inner poise and grace. This grace is the natural harmony of the Tao expressing itself.

Footprints on the Path

It is difficult to follow the path, and it is also difficult to be sure that we are on it. About this problem, Chuang Tzu, Lao Tzu's literary and spiritual successor, wrote: "If Tao could be explained, we would freely do so for our loved ones and our leaders. But it is not possible. Tao will not be found unless both inner and outer worlds are in harmony." This message, penned two hundred years after Lao Tzu, reiterates Lao Tzu's fundamental message.

Try as we might to define Tao, its true meaning will always escape intellectual explanation. All attempts to interpret Tao serve largely to confuse people. It cannot be found through words or through an intellectual quest. The effortless state of existence that is the epitome of finding Tao requires a return to nature and a corresponding abandonment of the social organizations that enslave us. Chuang Tzu explains this idea in the following passage:

"Tao is without beginning, without end. Other things are born and die. They are impermanent; and now for better, now for worse, they are ceaselessly changing form. Past years cannot be recalled; time cannot be arrested. The succes-

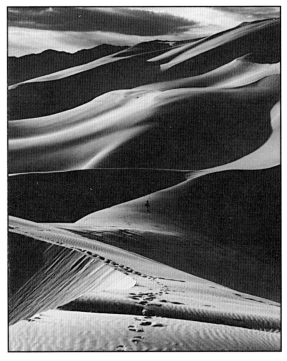

sion of states is endless, and every end is followed by a new beginning. Thus it may be said that a man's duty to his neighbor is embodied in the eternal principles of the universe. The life of man passes like a galloping horse, changing at every turn, at every hour. What should he do, or what should he not do, other than let his decomposition continue."

THE TANTRIC PRACTICE OF CHÖD

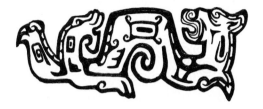

There are many esoteric practices that we can use to free ourselves of the sometimes overwhelming influences of our emotions. One of the most severe is the tantric practice of Chöd. It is used literally to destroy any emotional attachment we might have to our own bodies. After prayer, practitioners enter deep states of meditation and then begin the psychic sacrifice of their own body. The body, first envisioned as ugly and overweight, is then conceived of as the place where our hatreds and lusts reside. A wrathful goddess, personifying the wisdom mind, is then envisioned. Piece by piece, she is imagined cutting the body to shreds. Finally, the pieces of the corpse are thrown into a boiling pot. At this point, what is left of the body begins to radiate pure light that is then offered to all those in need of such energy, including the poor, the homeless, wandering animal spirits, and even demons. In this way, the practitioner becomes free of earthly attachment and the stultifying effect of uncontrolled emotions.

In one sense, such a formulation of the Tao seems, at first glance, to be deeply pessimistic in its suggestion that we have virtually no control over our lives. The sage implies that aspects of our lives that we desperately attempt to manage will always elude us. On the other hand, though, the truth of these words is completely self-evident. Ultimately they are able to inspire hope and even joy. The meaning of Chuang Tzu's message is this: There is no other recourse for us. What we must do in our lives is simply to be, nothing more.

Chuang Tzu also tells us how to identify those who exemplify the life of one who seeks the Tao. "The wise," he said, "are charitable, not from a sense of duty but because it is The Way. They do not acquire debt nor place others under obligation to them. They take their food where they may find it and they ramble carefree through the world." The wise are those who realize that nature and destiny cannot be changed. And they know that by virtue of being human, we, too, are part of nature.

Renouncing Society

This theme of seeking the Tao by departing from society is revisited often in Taoist poetry and art, and it is a central concept in Taoist thought. Chi K'ang, a Taoist poet of the 2nd century A.D., was likely young and romantic at the time of writing the following verses:

I will cast out Wisdom
  and reject Learning.
My thoughts shall wander
  in the Great Void
Always repenting of wrongs done
Will never bring my heart to rest.
I cast my hook in a single stream;
But my joy is as though
  I possessed a Kingdom.
I loose my hair and go singing;
To the four frontiers
  men join in my refrain.
This is the purport of my song:
"My thoughts shall wander
  in the Great Void."

Chi K'ang tells us that what we commonly think of as knowledge and wisdom are obstacles in his path. What he has learned, he realizes, will not help him in his contemplation of Tao. Furthermore, spending his time in regret and reflecting on the sins of his past will bring him neither peace nor enlightenment.

Fishing in the little stream is a metaphor he uses to refer to a life lived with the Tao. Communion with the Tao will provide him with all he needs—food and happiness fit for a king. By untying his hair, he symbolically frees himself from societal conventions. His song, reminding people of their spiritual obligation to the Tao, is like a signal that will awaken all who hear it.

Like other Taoists, the poet never really does tell us what the Tao is. He can only show us the direction in which he is looking for Tao and the virtue he finds in its seeking. This method of indi-

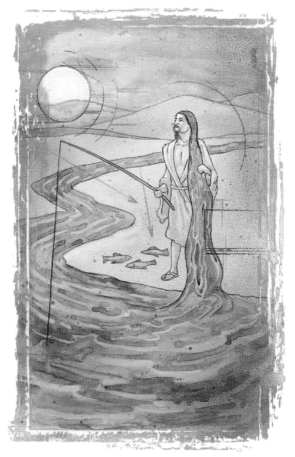

rectly discussing Tao is very much in keeping with the traditional Taoist path.

To the Taoist, an enlightened mind is a mind unencumbered with the intellectual constructions of society. Enlightenment is a state of mind in which the universal principles that govern nature are reflected without effort. Ideas born from such a state cannot help but surpass the more mundane ideas of an unenlightened mind. Unfortunately, simply being born into society has, as a consequence, the inheritance of its confusion. Religions, legal systems, and rituals are all examples of the contrived systems that serve the private interests of certain groups. When we adopt the ideas they propound, we also adopt their interests and ways of thinking. By doing so, we lose sight of the true nature of things. How best to rid ourselves of these misconceptions and flawed logic is the Taoist problem.

Our five senses are partly to blame because they encourage us to explore the outer world. At times we are led by our eyes, and at others we follow our ears on a fool's quest. The psychological effects of colors, sound, smell, taste, and physical sensations in general, therefore, must be carefully controlled. "The five colors blind our eyes, the five sounds deafen our ears, and the five flavors spoil our taste," says Lao Tzu in Verse 12 of the *Tao Te Ching*.

He implies that behind the world of the senses lies another world, an inner reality complete with its own sensibilities, all superior to our physical perceptions. Unfortunately, too much contact with the exterior world causes us to lose touch with that inner dimension and consequently with Tao. This idea of an inner world that requires our energy and attention is central to Taoist thought. Because our attention is distracted by the outer world, our energies are diverted

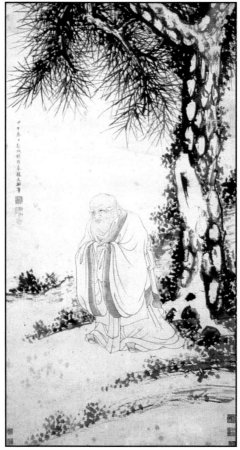

Lao Tzu, author of the *Tao Te Ching*

from the more important, inner tasks. As a result, we unnecessarily delay our return journey to the source, to the Tao.

As Lao Tzu says in Verse 47 of the *Tao Te Ching*:

> *One may know the world*
> * without going out of doors.*
> *One may know the Way*
> * of Heaven without looking*
> * through the windows.*
> *The further one goes,*
> * the less one knows.*
> *Therefore the sage knows*
> * without going about,*
> *Understands without seeing,*
> *And accomplishes without*
> * any action.*

The passage suggests that it is not the world as such that must be renounced, but rather its outer appearance. We can know the world, the passage tells us, without actually exploring it. By exploring it we never reach the heart of the world, but only meet its shell, the part that envelops it and conceals its true inner nature. The Way tells us to direct attention away from the overwhelming flood of ideas produced in our interaction with the everyday world. By doing so, it is possible to gain a measure of control over our emotions, since we no longer need to respond to the world. If we can accomplish this, then the messages we receive from the world, although endless in their scope, can no longer influence us in the same manner, nor can they determine our outlook.

In this way, Taoists believe our inner world will gradually be purified and liberated from both the tyranny of the senses and the radical swings of emotion they invoke. Freedom from the boundaries imposed by daily life now becomes possible. After progressing a certain distance on The Way, we escape the mundane laws affecting human existence. As our spirit develops, old patterns of thinking and behavior are left behind. This inner work of Taoism is not only about acquiring something new; it is about freeing ourselves from something damaging that we already have—the training we receive from society.

Artistic Expression of Taoism

Taoism has much in common with the philosophy espoused by the great Greek philosopher Socrates. The famous Socratic maxim, "Know thyself," is based on his belief that by searching inward, into the mind and its mysterious operations, the seeker will find a pure form of knowledge, untainted by outside influences. He theorized that an understanding and development of the psychological self *(continued on page 72)*

KNOWLEDGE TRAVELS NORTH

Chuang Tzu demonstrates many of the abstract and ambiguous qualities of Taoism in this wonderful excerpt from one of his stories entitled, "Knowledge Travels North."

"When Knowledge traveled north across the Black Water, and over the Dark-Steep Mountain, he met Do-nothing Say-nothing and asked of him as follows:

'Kindly tell me by what thoughts, by what cogitations, may Tao be known. By resting in what, by according in what, may Tao be approached? By following what, by pursuing what, may Tao be attained?'

To these three questions, Do-nothing Say-nothing returned no answer. Not that he would not answer, but that he could not. So when Knowledge got no reply, he turned round and went off to the south of the White Water and up the Ku-Chuen Mountain, where he saw All-in-extremes, and to him he put the same questions.

'Ha!' cried All-in-extremes, 'I know. I will tell you . . .'

But just when he was about to speak, he forgot what he wanted to say. So when Knowledge got no reply, he went back to the palace and asked the Yellow Emperor.

The latter said, 'By no thoughts, by no cogitations, Tao may be known. By resting in nothing, by according in nothing, Tao may be approached. By following nothing, by pursuing nothing, Tao may be attained.'

Then Knowledge said to the Yellow Emperor, 'Now you and I know this, but those two know it not. Who is right?'

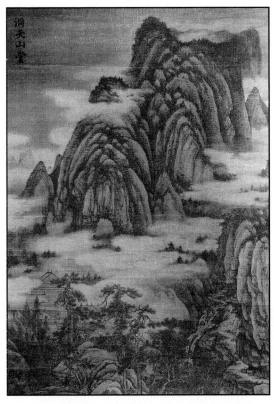

'Of those two', replied the Yellow Emperor, 'Do-nothing Say-nothing is genuinely right, and All-in-extremes is near. You and I are wholly wrong. Those who understand it do not speak about it, those who speak about it do not understand it.'"

would lead to a corresponding development of the soul. As we have seen, a similar idea plays an important role in Taoist thought.

Like modern day psychologists, the ancient Taoists came to realize that a set of deeply seated motivations underlie our daily actions. These motivating forces remain hidden, yet actively work to determine our behavior. In the modern world, we use many different techniques to explore those motivations. Through discussion and sometimes using supplementary techniques like hypnosis, dream analysis, or drugs, professional counselors attempt to uncover these forces.

Taoist teachers agree that as we age, we learn to accept certain ideas and beliefs about ourselves and others and about how the world works in general. Once we have accepted them, they become part of us, and we refuse to modify them even if they are absolutely wrong. Over time, these ideas sink to the back of our minds, and while they still influence our thinking processes, we are no longer aware they even exist. In this way, our hidden values can indeed determine our everyday patterns of thought and behavior.

The basic problem with these hidden values is that they are unnecessarily restricting and can even be dangerous. Eventually, they can manifest as a pathological condition. Unlike the clients of psychologists, however, practicing Taoists do not wait for an actual problem to develop before attempting to discover and modify the roots of their behavior. As part of their discipline, they naturally become aware of their hidden motivations. They are also well-aware that their discipline ultimately leads to self-transformation; it is a type of spiritual alchemy that enables practitioners to progress from an ordinary life to one more refined with many more possibilities.

Taoist practices seek to reduce these potentially damaging limitations in three realms of human concern: the physical, the psychological, and the spiritual. Interestingly, our limitations manifest in ways that correspond to these three realms. In terms of the physical, we learn to be inflexible and awkward in our movements. Over time, this state negates the natural athletic abilities most of us possess as children. Secondly, in terms of the psychological, we learn unhealthy and unproductive mental behaviors. For this reason, sloth is regarded in many cultures as a deadly sin. Finally, in terms of our spirit, we adopt negative, even cynical attitudes that not only stifle our own creativity and joy, but can lead to self-destruction and even the ruination of others.

Taoism is a practice devoted to casting off these limitations, many of that are learned through our social interactions. It is a self-imposed discipline that involves many procedures including, among others, chanting, meditation, and the physical movements of tai chi chuan. Some styles use ritual and prayer as well.

The Limitations of Language

When comparing Taoist and psychological approaches to the idea of self-transformation, one feature becomes very apparent: Many psychologi-

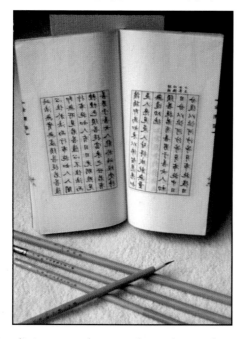

cal techniques, such as psychoanalysis, rely extensively on discussion as a methodology. Proponents of these psychological approaches hope that by recognizing the underlying motivating forces that lead to behavior, the client will actually be able to change the resulting behavior. This may or may not be true. Taoist practice, on the other hand, typically avoids conversation altogether, unless it is related to direct instruction. In Taoist practice, personal transformation is thought to result strictly from performing the prescribed exercises. The type of insight that results from therapeutic discussion is not highly valued.

The whole idea of the limitations of language and conversation when trying to express ideas relating to inner transformation has a very long history. Chuang Tzu, for example, noted the inadequacy of language in the attempt to express deep meaning. "The universe is very beautiful," he wrote, "yet it says nothing. The four seasons abide by a fixed law, yet they are not heard. All creation is based upon absolute principles, yet nothing speaks." Chuang Tzu is simply trying to point out that we can appreciate beauty and recognize wisdom and knowledge without discussing any of it.

As a result of this aversion to language as a tool for self-expression, Taoists learned to use other methods of self-expression. The art of calligraphy, for instance, seeks to express certain qualities using written symbols and exactly what is said is not the only important factor. The true beauty in calligraphy is found in the lettering itself. Advancing on the path is not so much an expression of meaning or even what is done, but of how things are expressed. The object of the discipline is found in its doing. This characteristic still holds true today.

In spite of these very different approaches to achieving inner transformation, the goals of psychologists and Taoist teaching masters are similar. They seek to help others reach a state of inner balance. Taoists have traditionally believed that it is far easier to show the path to Tao than it is to explain it. They prefer to inspire seekers through literature, artwork, or demonstration, letting imagery and metaphor convey their message. Certain media lend themselves more favorably to the expression of Taoist ideas than others.

Typically, the ideas of Taoism have been expressed in painting, poetry, fables, legends, and even in medicine and the martial arts. Since it is an inherent truth of Taoism that nothing very definite can ever be said about it, Taoist ideas have assumed a secretive and enigmatic character over the centuries. Rich in description and metaphor, set in natural scenes of forests and lakes, often including birds and other animals, Taoist writings and other art forms conjure up many meanings, often deeply personal to the reader. Although Taoist writing can sometimes be abstract and philosophical, these works are always characterized by a certain ambiguity that leaves room for the reader to reflect on its meaning.

Taoism: The Invisible Force Behind the Chinese Arts

Even though Taoist ideas took hold in mainstream Chinese thought and are now deeply rooted, the historical effects of its presence are in some ways difficult to trace. In the second century B.C., the historian Ss-ma Ch'ien noted that

MAKING THE INK

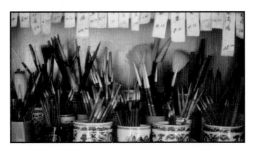

The brush, brush stand, ink, and grinding stone are referred to as the "Four Treasures of the Literature Room." Since these tools are essential to the work of students, painters, and calligraphers alike, the four treasures are found in every study. Each of the four is completely dependent on the others. Without one, the rest are useless. Over time, each article has been invested with many layers of symbolic meaning, and each has a long and venerable history. The process of making ink is one example.

Making ink is a painstaking process. Since it is made from carbon, the first step is to select the wood, usually either fir or pine. Then it is slowly burned at just the right temperature in the furnace for many days. Later the residual carbon is scraped from the sides and mixed with a glue. The compound is then shaped into sticks or blocks and left to harden. This substance is later mixed with water and ground by the artist to make ink as it is required. Early ink mixtures often contained powdered jade, a substance considered by the Chinese to be very precious. Taoists were particularly fond of jade and considered it to be the food of the spirits.

the Taoist teachings of Chuang Tzu were like flood waters that knew no boundaries and could not be contained. The irony is that in spite of its popularity, no one, not even the rulers or professional administrators themselves, could find any specific application for Taoism. Surely this was the intention of Chuang Tzu.

For whatever reason, since the fifth century, serious Chinese scholars have rejected the Taoist ideas of Chuang Tzu. The reverse is true, however, of poets, of landscape painters, and curiously enough, of Zen Buddhists. In these disciplines, his influence has been extremely dramatic. At the core of these disciplines his Taoist ideals still thrive.

We have seen how Taoist concepts do not lend themselves well to certain kinds of investigations. Lao Tzu has made it clear enough that the Tao cannot be known through intellectual analysis. Chuang Tzu has made it clear that the Tao can only be known in a visionary way. Tu Meng of the Tang Dynasty (618–905), in one of his 120 aphorisms relating to calligraphy, explains: "A divine work is not achieved through human understanding but through intuition."

However, visual and poetic images readily lend themselves to the expression of Tao. Although these arts are often profound in their expressive ability, they are not encumbered by the restrictions of intellectual content. Looking at the ideas behind Taoist painting and in the fine art of calligraphy, then, is a good place to begin.

Chinese painting was not traditionally considered to be a profession. Instead, its practice was believed to indicate a certain degree of maturity on the part of the painter. Paintings were regarded as something of a synthesis of the individual's life accomplishments. Many past masters of Chinese painting first achieved prominence in other professions before taking up the brush.

Chinese painting is associated with an immense literature that includes, among other fields, history, religion, poetry, and philosophy. In this literature there are many signs of Taoist influence. In the past, aspiring artists trained in all of these fields simply to become acquainted with the ideas and their associated symbols. As a result, in China the painter is very often a philosopher and poet as well as a professional of some other type.

But a great Chinese artist is not developed simply through the mastery of formal style alone. It requires spiritual development as well. Li Jih-hua (1565–1635) eloquently describes the habits of a great painter in the following passage:

> When Huang Tzuchiu meditates
> he sits alone in the wilds,
> with only the bamboos, the trees
> and scrub and the rocks for
>   company.
> Others do not understand him,
> for he is not a part of their world.

Every now and then
he travels to the confluence
of the great river and the sea.
There, he rests, in the wind and rain
amidst furious water spirits.
Such is the heart and soul
of the Great Absent Minded
  (his nickname).
In his solidarity with the elements
lies a secret—his magnificent works
  reflect
the ever-changing moods and
  feelings of Nature
and so, become truly great.

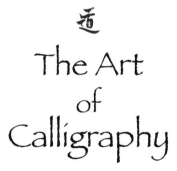

The Art
of
Calligraphy

Calligraphy is an art related to Chinese painting since it, too, uses brush and ink. It is the practice of forming lines on paper in a particular way. At its highest level, it is the art of expressing inner understanding. The lines created by a calligrapher are known as characters and each one symbolically represents an idea or even a part of an idea. These lines are the Asian counterpart to the

Western alphabet. While there are many differences between the Western and Asian systems of writing, one of central importance is that to the calligrapher an idea is expressed not only by the character itself but in the quality of its execution. Exactly how the character is created is of para-

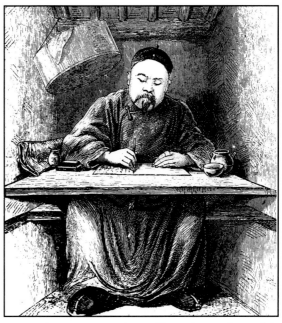

mount importance. For calligraphers, then, this quest for the formation of ideal characters is deeply personal.

The key to success in this discipline lies in being close to Tao. Proper composition of a line is simply not possible unless the inner being of the calligrapher is also perfectly composed. Here again, we see the idea of an inner, psychological world corresponding with the outer world. Over time, critics of calligraphy have pinpointed a number of major shortcomings found in beginning students. The weaknesses are reflections of the students' inner being. And so, the exercise is

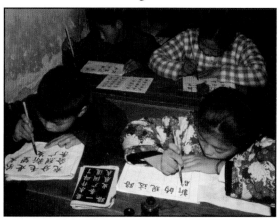

for students to develop internally to the point where the weaknesses are replaced by strengths. Together the defects are known as Pa-Ping, or "The Eight Defects." Since these are common to all, identifying them can help students with Tao. Critics of calligraphy rely on four categories for their analysis. For example, a character is said to possess varying degrees of bone, flesh, muscle, and blood. When these qualities are in the right proportions, the work is living. It expresses Tao. How better to evaluate the composition of a character than to compare it with something alive and healthy?

Each character, for example, must demonstrate inner strength, known as bone. It must also have the correct proportion of flesh so that it is neither too fat nor lean. Its blood (a quality related to the amount of water mixed with the ink) must be healthy in color. The quality of muscle in the work is left for the viewer to decide. In this way, the calligrapher's work becomes an expression of life itself. How is it that there are so many rules and such rigorous discipline in an art that seeks to express the inexpressible naturally? Such is the mystery of the Tao.

Meditation and the Mortar and Pestle

It is a compelling sight to watch students mix their ink in preparation for painting. Sitting cross-legged in front of little wooden tables, dressed in their robes, they make the ink. The ink is in the shape of a stick, and together with some water, it is mixed in a small circular container made from slate. The substance is very gradually ground up and made first into a paste and then finally into a smooth, flowing liquid. Immersed in their task, the artists pay no attention whatsoever to onlookers. Deep in meditation, they are totally oblivious to outside distraction. Beginners in calligraphy are often instructed to contemplate the work they are about to imitate. Those more advanced simply empty their minds.

Such is the intensity and depth of concentration required in Chinese brush painting. More than simply a preparation of the materials, grinding the ink is a time-honored tradition. It is a form of meditation and so, by preparing the ink, the artist is also preparing personally. By watching

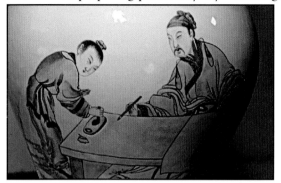

someone prepare in this fashion, it is possible to steal a glimpse of Tao.

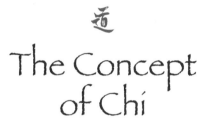

The Concept of Chi

Sometime around 500 A.D., a portrait painter named Hsieh Ho wrote a treatise describing the six essential points of a fine painting. His work is a cornerstone in the art of Chinese brush painting. The six ideas can be summarized in the following way:

> The movement of the Chi
> produces the movement of life.
> The brush brings structure
> into being.

Study an object before
   drawing its form.
Study its inner qualities
   before applying color.
Assign the elements of painting
   to their most suitable places.
When practicing and copying
   the work of a past master,
   be certain to transmit
   the inner qualities as
   well as the outer form.

In these few lines, we see several ideas: the concept of chi, the ability to observe inner essence, the idea of perfect balance, the idea of the essence of an object, and the notion of observing before acting—all very prominent in Taoist thought. Firstly, there is the underlying theme of meaning as it is expressed in the essence of a work. A Taoist painter, like other types of Taoist artists, must learn to see the inner nature of the subject. A Taoist martial artist does exactly the same thing with the opponent. Accomplishing this requires an understanding of chi, a special force existing in all things.

Secondly, Hsieh Ho associates the idea of chi, meaning vital force or breath of life, with a worthy painting. A work with chi is "living" in the sense that this primal vitality can actually be seen in the work. According to Taoist doctrine, chi is found throughout the cosmos, and it is the animating force and sustaining principle behind all living things. The concept of chi, of fundamental importance to Taoist practice, will be discussed at length in later chapters. But the idea of chi is relied on extensively in all Taoist arts, and it assumes particular importance in the practice of traditional Chinese medicine and in the martial arts.

Cultivating the Chi

While Taoists are not always able to describe the Tao, they did, and still do, have very specific sets of instructions as to how it might be attained. "Cultivating the chi" is one of those practices. The phrase refers to the practice of strengthening our personal life force. Once it is developed, it then can be applied to any task at hand, such as a brush stroke, a healing touch, or a forceful blow. Regardless of the application, chi exercises are well known in all disciplines with Taoist and Buddhist origins. True to the tradition, chi exercises do not have an intellectual character, but instead focus on a special type of physical discipline that sometimes involves meditation and mental imagery. Here Taoism leaves the domain of philosophy and enters the realm of mysticism, because to the untrained person, chi is an invisible and intangible force. Without special training, it cannot in any way be detected. Still, the idea of chi lies close to the heart of Taoist studies.

While we cannot with any great success capture the essence of Tao in a systematic, intellectual manner, we can describe our particular relationship with the Tao. As we have seen, certain forms of communication, particularly speechless forms like brush painting and tai chi chuan, but also literary works such as poetry and parable, are more eloquent than others.

道

The Idea of Mastery

"Taoist Master" is a term of respect reserved for those who are close to the Tao. Usually this accomplishment takes the better part of a lifetime. The few who do reach the Tao are individuals who understand The Way as far as any of us are able. Until recently, at least, there has been a reluctance on the part of these masters to commit their teachings to writing. Some simply have not believed that it was possible to do with any degree of exactitude. Others have felt uncomfortable passing this knowledge on to the general public. A few have worried that the information would fall into the wrong hands. As Taoism spread, different sects adopted different practices, and many branches sprang up. Even now, each group has specific policies about passing on information. Some sects guarded their inner practices as they might a treasure chest. In fact, so closely did they watch over their ideas that even today many of their methods are concealed.

Two of the most secretive groups of all were the Taoist alchemists and those who practiced tai chi chuan. While secrecy may protect and preserve knowledge, it also has the effect of generating misunderstanding. Because of their reluctance to discuss their ideas with outsiders, a great deal of confusion has surrounded these Taoist groups. One important misconception concerns the actual purpose of the practice of alchemy. Typically when speaking of alchemy, the idea of transmuting base metals into gold springs to mind. Nothing could be further from the truth.

Like their western counterparts, the Chinese alchemists were far more interested in discovering the secrets of long life, perfect health, superior knowledge, the cultivation of spirit, and even immortality than in the conversion of base metal to gold. In fact, it has been suggested that the language of the alchemists and the whole idea of transmuting metals was developed to mislead anyone who inadvertently overheard a Taoist conversation or read one of their treatises.

Preservation of Knowledge

Secrecy is also very much a part of the history of tai chi chuan, although the methods for preserving secrets were somewhat different. In many schools, certain instructions were never revealed until, perhaps after a lifetime of dedica-

THE SPREAD OF ALCHEMY

In its earliest form, alchemy likely originated in ancient Egypt. At that time it was devoted largely to metallurgy, and it was predominantly concerned with refining metals, particularly gold and silver, into purer substances. The residual matter from these processes was said to contain wonderful properties. These associations were, no doubt, the beginning of the later quest for immortality so often associated with these first chemists.

Later, these techniques developed into full-fledged metallurgic science. From these practices, bronze casting techniques also developed, and the reputation of the Egyptians as skilled metal workers spread across the Mediterranean Sea to Greece. After the conquest of Egypt by the Arabs, the methods spread to Spain, where they were developed to an even more specific science. The word alchemy itself may have come into existence when the Arabs attached the article, "al," meaning "the" to the word "kemya" meaning "chemistry." From Spain, the science spread throughout Europe.

Alchemy has had three central concerns over the centuries. These are the transmutation of base metals into finer substances, the quest for immortality, and the creation of artificial life forms known as Homunculi. In the nineteenth century, European alchemists banded together and assumed the name of the Hermetic Association. Organizations such as this one may continue even today.

tion, the master would condescend to entrust one or two of the most worthy students. A similar phenomenon occurs in yogic practice, where a yogi will teach two curricula, one for the general public and one for the inner circle of dedicated students. In the first half of this century, for example, tai chi chuan was a little known art even in China itself. Very few practiced it, and literature on the subject could not be found. This scarcity was not accidental; it reflected the teaching methods of the masters. Still, in a civilization abundant with literary works of all descriptions, it was highly unusual that almost nothing could be found on one of the civilization's greatest achievements. As an unfortunate consequence of this predisposition for secrecy, the Taoist arts came to be known derogatorily as "Taoist magic tricks," and "reputable" philosophers turned their attention elsewhere.

As we have suggested, there were some notable exceptions to this silence, and writings pertinent to Taoist discoveries could be found in the fields of medicine, literature, and art. Throughout these texts, the terms Tao (The Way), yin (feminine) and yang (masculine), chi (life force), jing (essence), and shen (spirit), to name only a few, appear with conspicuous regularity. Over the centuries, these ideas have been the subject of investigation by a variety of artists working in many different disciplines. As a result, Taoist art can today be thought of as a distinct school, complete with unique methods, favorite tools, typical themes, and underlying philosophy.

It is the work of all Taoists whether they are painters, poets, or martial artists, to develop their understanding of Tao, to develop a sense of The Way. In some cases, Taoists feel it necessary to express this relationship in a form that can be shared with others. This can be a difficult task since Taoist ideas are at best elusive and in many ways defy description, whether verbal or artistic. Nevertheless, it can be done. With its clean, suggestive images, made with the simple tools of brush and ink, for example, traditional Chinese painting has long sought to preserve The Way.

But for the student of the Tao, the study of the effects of the yang of action and the yin of inaction is all-consuming. How we act, what we say and do, our everyday thoughts and most secret motivations, combine to form our being. Equally important is what we do not say and do not do. Studying ourselves and others in this way leads us to an inevitable conclusion: How we conduct ourselves in the world is a reflection of what we have become internally. Knowing this is knowing Tao.

Chi and its applications

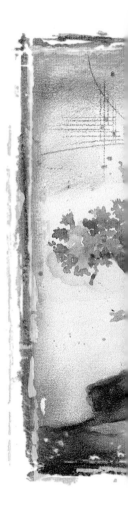

氣

Ancient Chinese myths and legends have told us about the Tai Chi and about Tao. They have also introduced us to a mysterious force, a primal substance that animates the universe. This substance is known as chi. It is the force that sets the world and everything in it into motion. Chi is also the force that sustains all things once they are created.

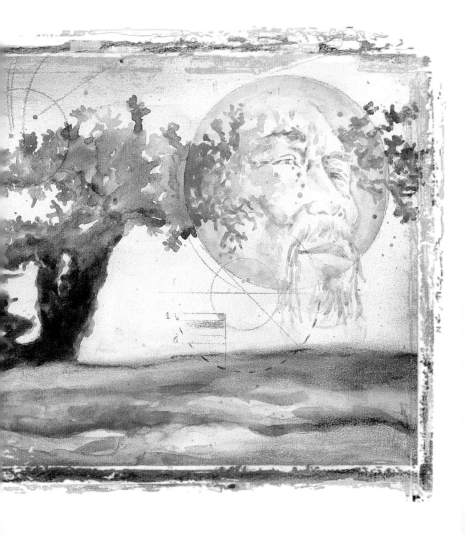

氣
The Idea of Chi

The idea of chi is not easily accepted by Westerners. It is not a concept that appears in our mainstream religions or philosophies. Neither do our medical and scientific traditions acknowledge chi or even have any place for it in their theories. In China and the Orient, however, the concept of chi is very familiar, even commonplace. Everyone, from politicians to school children, understands it. The notion of chi and its applications are as much a part of Chinese life and outlook as are the ideas of muscle tone and physical fitness in Western life.

Easterners believe chi to be the life energy contained within matter. In experiments conducted in the 1960s, nuclear physicists in China came to accept the notion that chi is actually a low-frequency, highly concentrated form of infrared radiation. In the last decade, experiments in China have been conducted on this special type of energy. Some researchers have come to believe, just as the legends tell us, that certain people may be able to learn to emit this form of energy from their bodies. Known as chi kung masters, these highly trained individuals often devote their lives to developing this subtle energy.

As the concept of chi crossed over into the West in recent years, a Western word was coined to describe it. Since chi has a number of properties that seem similar to those of electrical energy, it is sometimes called bio-energy. This describes the living energy that is native to life rather than to the inanimate forces of nature such as water power or lightning. Knowledge related to bio-energy is called bio-information.

The "Life Force"

However one conceives of chi, there is general agreement about what it does: Chi animates matter, infusing it with life. As a result, it is often described as the "life force." It not only permeates the empty spaces between material objects, it is part of their composition. In people and animals, for example, chi is responsible for the functioning of the organs, including the cardio-respiratory system. It circulates throughout the body with the blood so that it can provide its own particular form of nutrition to the myriad cells.

Every living organism has some way to assimilate chi. Human beings, animals, and plants alike ingest it along with the air they breathe, the water they drink, and the food they eat. Once inside, chi moves to various locations and begins to perform its many functions. The most common of these functions are generally related to the proper functioning and continued operation of the body or plant.

There are hints here and there in our culture that we in the Western world once did recognize

the mysterious force called chi. Have you ever
wondered, for example, why a mother kisses her
child's wound to try and make it better? It's
remarkable that after her kiss, the pain does often

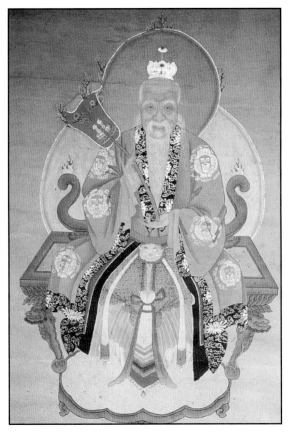

vanish. Psychologists may tell you this phenomenon has nothing to do with the kiss itself. Its
effectiveness, they say, is a result of the suggestion placed in the child's mind: The pain disappears as a result of a type of hypnosis induced by

the mother. But anyone who understands chi will say that the mother passed some of her life force into the child's damaged tissue. The life force not only repairs the wound, it also serves as an anesthetic.

Another example can be found in many of the devotional paintings created by our finest artists. In these works, you can often find a halo surrounding the heads of Christ, the Madonna, the disciples, visiting angels, cherubs, and many other members of the heavenly host. Some believe this aura to be simply a fanciful symbol created by the artist for effect. Others, however, believe they can actually see these emanations radiating from holy people and others who have cultivated the chi to a high degree. Some gifted artists, who were especially sensitive to color and light, may have taken their inspiration for the idea of halos directly from a particularly radiant person.

Experiencing Chi: An Experiment

Most people are understandably skeptical about this energy until they actually experience it for themselves. After all, in the West we have been well trained to deny even the possibility of such phenomena. While some people will never be able to sense the chi, many others do—some on their first encounter with it.

Try this experiment with a partner, such as your child, spouse, or friend, to see if you are able

THE AMAZING FORCE OF CHI

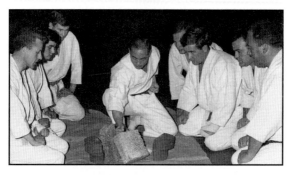

For a really compelling demonstration of the applications of chi, visit a well-known martial arts training studio on a night when it is giving demonstrations to the public. Known as a dojo, such a studio teaches people of all ages and abilities about the mental and physical disciplines related to the various martial arts. On special demonstration nights, the students, in their best dress, will proudly demonstrate their skills. Typically these presentations offer sparring competitions between students of similar ages and abilities. The master presides and usually observes silently from a strategic position. On some nights, more advanced students and their instructors perform stunning feats.

Make sure you attend on a night when these demonstrations as well as sparring competitions are given. Everyone has heard of feats such as breaking bricks with the fists, forehead, and palm. But how about breaking just the middle brick alone in a stack? Martial artists claim to do these sorts of things with their chi.

to feel the chi. Both of you should either sit or stand approximately two arms-length away from each other. Ask your partner to close his eyes and take a deep breath. Relax your shoulders and back muscles as completely as possible. Try to imagine an energy rising from the ground into your body.

When you think you can almost sense this imaginary force, ask your partner to extend an arm toward you until it is level with the floor. The palm of the hand should be facing downward. Slowly raise your own arms and extend your fingers until they are within a few inches of your partner's outstretched hand. Using your mind, direct the imaginary energy—what we call the chi. Move it further up through your body until it passes along your arms and out from your fingertips. It's helpful to imagine a current of energy passing from your body into your partner's. Whether you think this is an imaginary force or not, some people feel the chi right away, even with their eyes closed.

More powerful demonstrations of the application of chi can be found in Chinese medical centers, where acupuncture techniques are used on patients ready to undergo surgery. The acupuncture is used to stimulate the chi, which then induces anesthesia. Using these techniques, patients regularly undergo major operations without drugs. *(See Chapter 5, "Traditional Chinese Medicine," for more about acupuncture.)*

THERAPEUTIC TOUCH AND CHI

Over the last twenty years, a new course in treatment has been introduced to Western medical students. The course has been added to the nursing curriculum at as many as eighty univer-

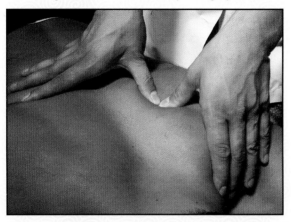

sities around the world. It is designed around a healing technique that has been used for hundreds, perhaps thousands, of years. This skill, called "therapeutic touch," has taken the nursing profession by storm. It is based on the ancient practice of "laying on of hands," a healing art that dates back to ancient times and was first documented long ago in the form of early cave wall pictographs. Written accounts of this healing technique appear later in the Bible. The idea behind the practice is simple: A practitioner simply places his hands on the client and emits life-energy into their body.

Interestingly enough, the idea of rediscovering such a simple healing system from ancient times is often disturbing to Westerners, who are more familiar with and therefore more comfortable with a strictly scientific approach to healing. But in China and many other Asian countries, healers have never ceased to recognize the importance of this life energy in the dynamic workings of the human body. In fact, they rely on it. This force is chi, the very same form of energy we have been discussing.

Therapeutic touch begins when the healer centers himself, directing his attention. Next, the healer assesses the energy field of the patient. Using the palms of his hands, he "feels" the flow of energy by passing his hands over the body, although he never actually touches it. As part of their training, practitioners learn to develop many levels of this energy-sensing ability and apply them in their work.

As the healer continues to work with the patient, the energy fields of both the practitioner and the client "mesh." This allows the healer to effect a change in the client and transform or move the energy field toward a more balanced state.

In the next chapter, we will discuss the Chinese art known as chi kung, a healing practice often used in traditional Chinese medicine. You will see the remarkable similarity between these two arts.

Chi: The Vital Force

Chi is a special substance with certain properties. As it has traditionally been understood, it refers to a vital force, the animating force behind life itself, and has always been associated with both breath and air. A more contemporary view sees chi as a substance much like light, with properties of both matter and energy. Some, such as chi kung masters, claim to be able to project chi from their bodies into others and to be able to see it. In fact, the chi may be the healing substance responsible for the phenomenon known as the "laying on of hands." This is a healing tradition known in the West in which one or more people will place their hands on someone who is not well. Sometimes these people recover completely for reasons unknown to modern medicine.

Understanding the idea of chi requires us to recognize the extent of its influence both inside our bodies and in the world around us. The concept of chi, then, can be discussed in terms of how it appears in the universe and what it does.

In Taoist theory, both chi and Tao in their original forms are invisible and beyond the realm of normal human senses. Nevertheless, chi is found at the root of all movement, all change, and all things whether or not they are living.

Earlier, in the myth of Pan Ku, we saw how the One, in the form of an egg, gave birth to the two—the forces of yin and yang—and how Pan Ku was the third of the forces created. Lao Tsu, in Verse 42 of the *Tao Te Ching*, tells us that the Tao was responsible not only for these initial three creations, but also for everything created subsequently:

> Tao produced the One.
> The One produced the two.
> The two produced the three.
> And the three produced the ten
>   thousand things.
> The ten thousand things carry the yin
>   and embrace the yang, and through
>   the blending of the material force (ch'i)
>   they achieve harmony.

The verse tells us that the permutations of the yin and the yang and their interactions with the material force known as the chi produced the rest of creation, known figuratively in Chinese myth, folklore, and philosophy as the ten thousand things.

The chi referred to in this verse is found throughout the universe, on the most remote stars, in the tiniest speck of dust, and on the deepest ocean floors, in fact, in each of the ten thousand things. When this chi is identified in material bodies, it is given distinct names. In the human body alone, Chinese traditional physicians and chi kung practitioners have identified many forms of it, including prenatal chi, primary chi, pectoral chi, nutritional chi, and defensive chi. In nature, too, there are terms for different types of chi. These help us to distinguish among its many forms. But ultimately, all derive from their common source, known as universal chi.

In this sense, then, chi, a material force, acts as the agent of Tao, an immaterial force. We know that Tao was formless because in Verse 25 Lao Tsu, the acknowledged authority in these matters, tells us:

> There was something undifferentiated
>   and yet complete,
> Which existed before heaven and earth.
> Soundless and formless, it depends on
>   nothing and does not change.
> It operates everywhere and is free from
>   danger.
> It may be considered the mother of the
>   universe.
> I do not know its name; I call it Tao.

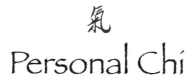

Personal Chi

Certain types of chi are naturally found within the human body. This natural chi is known as "personal," or "normal," chi. Personal chi is a general, umbrella term for the four primary forms of human chi. There are many different names for these four types, but they are commonly known as prenatal chi, nutritional chi, defensive chi, and pectoral chi. Their names reflect their functions within the body, each of which is described on the following pages.

Prenatal Chi: A Gift from our Parents

Prenatal chi, sometimes called primary chi, is transmitted directly to the child by the parents at the time of conception. This chi initially locates in and around the kidneys. As the organs of the body begin to function autonomously, the prenatal chi moves into the rest of the body. The quality of prenatal chi determines, in part, our general constitution—whether we are strong and healthy or weak and sickly. As we progress through life, we draw upon this chi, first to develop and grow, and then just to survive. Since there is a finite amount, we gradually exhaust the supply, and our bodies begin to deteriorate.

After birth, prenatal chi must be nourished by the food we eat, the water we drink, and the air we breathe. Since chi is a primordial substance of the body even more basic than blood, we must nourish it in order to nourish our bodies. The quality of the food and water we consume and the air we breathe has a direct effect on the quality of our prenatal chi. Once inside our system, food, water, and air are immediately transformed into unique types of chi. Each of these have special functions. Our health, then, is directly related

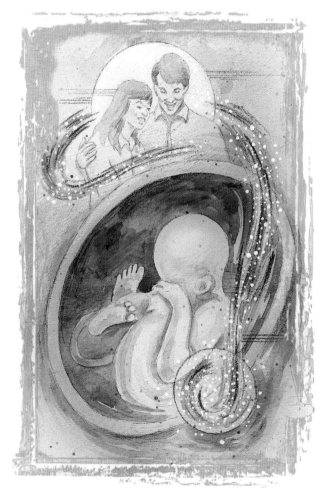

not only to the caliber of the chi transmitted to us at the time of our birth, but also to the quality of our food and air supplies. This means that the strength of our prenatal chi does not entirely dictate our destiny. Even if our prenatal chi is weak, we can still improve our chances of living a long and healthy life.

Nutritional Chi

There are several types of "acquired chi," which enter the body after birth. One of these is known as nutritional chi, and as mentioned above, it is created from the food we ingest. Produced by the spleen and stomach, it circulates in the blood vessels. Nutritional chi is responsible for producing the blood itself and also for providing the body with nourishment.

When it is found in the human body, chi and blood have always been understood to have a close association. An old Chinese expression says that chi is the commander of blood, but blood is the mother of chi. This means that wherever chi is to be found, the blood will follow.

On the other hand, it is the blood that nourishes the chi. This is one of the core ideas in traditional Chinese medicine. By increasing the amount of chi in deficient areas, the blood, because of its natural affinity to chi, will follow. This brings additional nutrients, moisture, and a fresh supply of oxygen to the damaged tissue. At the same time, the blood will nourish the existing chi. From this example, you can clearly see the give-and-take relationship, the yin and the yang at play, between the two substances.

Defensive Chi

Defensive chi also originates with the food we eat. Rather than flowing through the interior of the body as does the nutritional chi, its native habitat is close to the surface of the body, where it protects us against disease. It also is responsible for the operation of the pores, providing moisture to skin tissue and hair, and when necessary, helping to regulate body temperature.

Pectoral Chi

The air that we breathe is transformed into another type of chi known as natural air chi, or pectoral chi, after its location in the body. It enables the lungs to control respiratory functions and enables the heart to circulate the blood. This chi is also associated with the ability to move the limbs and trunk of the body and to circulate the chi in the body. People without stamina, and those who are unable to speak clearly or whose voices lack force, are said to be deficient in natural air chi.

氣

Seeing Is Believing

One simple but very convincing feat that demonstrates the power and presence of chi is known as "weight underside." This demonstration does not rely on physical strength, so even those who are relatively small in stature but familiar with the technique can give a very convincing performance. Two strong men stand on

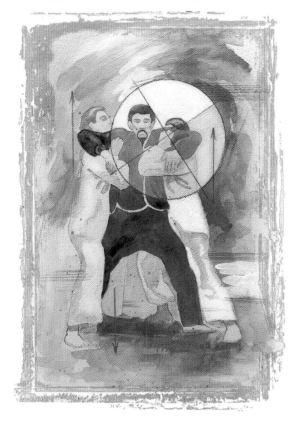

either side of the practitioner, each holding one arm, which is bent at the elbow and parallel to the floor. The bend in the arm makes a convenient supporting frame so the men have excellent leverage. Try as they might, after the initial preparation, the men will not be able to move the master, no matter how much force they use. It quickly

CONCENTRATING THE CHI

Accomplishing the weight underside tech-nique has much to do with an age-old Taoist practice of concentrating the chi in the abdomi-nal region at a point known as the tan tien. *This point is also called the* hara *by Japanese practitioners and the* shimen *or stone gate by acupuncturists. Tai chi chuan practitioners and many different types of martial artists are taught very early on in their training to direct the chi, using the mind, from the upper parts of the body to this point. Once the chi begins to concentrate here, it can then be mentally direct-ed to other locations both inside the body and outside.*

To describe to the practitioner the intricacy of moving the chi mentally through the body, the tai chi classic, The Mental Elucidation of the Thirteen Postures, *written by an unknown author, says "Let the chi move as if through a pearl with nine passageways. There is no part of the body the chi cannot reach." As a point of interest, a nine-channeled pearl is a wooden ball with nine intersecting channels in its interior. Young Chinese girls exercise with this ball to improve their manual dexterity. They practice moving a thread through the nine openings and along the channels without either breaking or tangling it.*

becomes a comical sight—two burly fellows looking desperate and shifting positions in a hopeless effort to move one average-size person from the standing position.

Such a feat cannot be accomplished without special knowledge of the chi. The secret is using the mind to direct the chi, which is used to "move" body weight to an imaginary location somewhere beneath the surface of the floor. As a result, the practitioner becomes virtually immovable. Once the central concepts are learned, masters say the exercise is quite easy to accomplish with regular practice. Using the mind to direct the chi is one of the central ideas in many of the martial arts, and it is particularly important to tai chi chuan. By training the mind in this way, practitioners can perform many astounding feats.

Weight underside is only one of many applications for chi. Other convincing demonstrations of the power of chi are related not only to combat but also to the healing arts. Chi is commonly used to relieve pain and stiffness of limbs and joints, to induce sleep, and to promote the healing of damaged organs or other body tissues. Advanced practitioners believe that when the chi circulates freely through the body, it can awaken latent psychic abilities. Some are able to absorb chi from the world around them and later emit it as a powerful radiation. Demonstrations of the power of chi are often given at various gatherings in Chinese communities.

THE SIX EVIL CHI

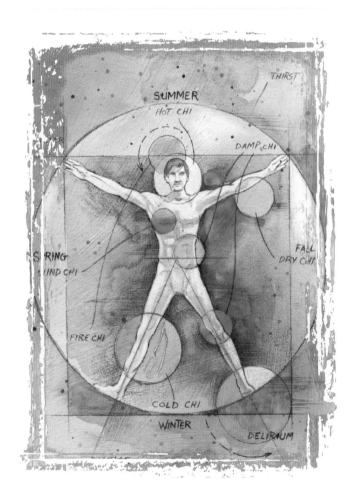

Chi not only manifests in living creatures, but it is also present throughout the inorganic world. Sometimes this chi from nature proves too powerful for the human body and illness can result. When this occurs, the chi is said to be "evil." Chinese physicians often warn their clients about the dangers to health associated with the natural environment. Over time, each of the different seasons has acquired a negative association with a particular kind of chi. Together these forces are known as the six evil chi.

Winter is associated with cold chi. When this external chi of the season moves inside a person, it is known as "internal cold," and it is treated as a disease. It is thought to be the cause of such problems as poor circulation, chills, headaches, and cramps. This ability to "attack" an individual is also true of the five other evil chi forces, and all of them produce their own unique diseases.

Hot chi is associated with summer and can cause excessive sweating and thirst, fevers, headaches, and sore throats. Damp chi is a property of late summer and causes sore joints, loss of appetite, and nausea.

Dry chi, native to fall, produces dry, cracked skin, dry coughs, and exhaustion. It is caused by insufficient moisture in the air and is especially harmful to the lungs.

The wind chi of spring is particularly nasty, and it is believed to affect the upper body parts first, including the lungs. Wind chi is traditionally considered to be the mother of all disease.

A final category, fire chi, is related to both the seasons and to emotional disorders. It is responsible for a number of problems including delirium, fevers, and inflammations. Any of the chi associated with the seasons, if they become extreme, can be transformed into fire chi.

Chi and Breathing

Knowledge of chi is not today, and never has been, exclusive to China. The idea that chi is an "intelligent" energy that protects the body and coordinates its functions has appeared in many cultures. This "living energy" is called *prana* in India, and in fact it very likely has been studied in that country for a longer period of time than in China itself. In his book *The Hindu-Yogi Science of Breath,* Yogi Ramacharaka succinctly describes prana:

"Prana is the name by which we designate a universal principle, which is the essence of all motion force or energy, whether manifested in gravitation, electricity, the revolution of the planets, and all forms of life, from the highest to the lowest. This great principle is in all forms of matter, and yet it is not matter. It is in the air, but it is not air nor one of its chemical constituents. Animal and plant life breathe it in with the air, and yet if they contained it not they would die even though they might be filled with air."

The notion that chi is related to breath was a favorite theme of the Indian sages of the Vedic Period. (*Veda* means wisdom in Sanskrit, the holy language of ancient India.) During this historical period, which began nearly four thousand years ago, the ancient sages began to record their ideas in written form. Many texts from the Vedic Period have been preserved to this day. Studying this literature, we realize that the idea of relating chi and breath is as old as time itself. In Sanskrit, prana means "ultimate energy," and when used in context with living organisms, it is recognized

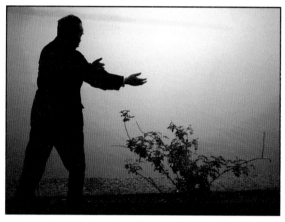

as the "vital animating force" in living things. Ever since that time, practitioners have believed that it was necessary to breathe to acquire this force, so the intimate relationship between the act of breathing and staying alive and well was established in this way. Consequently, innumerable breathing exercises from many different sects were developed specifically to increase the amount of available chi and to use it for special purposes.

Exactly who these ancient sages might have been, no one knows. The only traces of them are found in the Vedic literature and perhaps in some of the yogic practices. Their legacy, however, offers a wealth of information on topics related to the vital force in human life and how it may be purified. They observed in their incomparably poetic way, for example, that the basic emotions, such as fear, passion, rage, and anxiety, would cause corresponding physiological responses, all negative. The yogis, who later followed these secret teachings, noticed that these physical states were invariably related to, among other things, heart rate, muscular tension, and respiratory rate, and that undesirable mental states, such as confusion and disorientation, accompanied these changes.

The Benefits of Breathing Control

Breathing control, as it turned out, was central to their success in regulating these physiological responses. By controlling such variables as the volume of air, the rate at which it is inhaled and exhaled, the timing between the inhale and exhale, and the location in the lungs in which the air is placed, they could affect both mental and physical states of being. Using carefully prescribed breathing patterns, the masters learned to induce special states, such as deep meditation or heightened awareness, for use in specific situations. As a result of their painstaking research over the course of centuries, the masters made exciting discoveries related to health, strength, longevity, and even happiness. These ideas were systematized and became a basic part of the many different systems of psycho-physical exercises such as yoga. It was during this period of research that the relationship between breath and chi was firmly established.

It seems there is considerable truth to the hypothesis that special breathing techniques can indeed enhance certain functions of the body. It is well known, for example, that children with weak respiratory systems may be able to overcome their deficiencies if given a wind instrument to practice at a young age. The idea is that the act of exercising the lungs consistently over long periods of time will strengthen the muscle groups responsible for respiratory functions and increase the supply of oxygen to the entire body. According to traditional Chinese medical theory, by strengthening their breathing, children will increase the quantity of available pectoral chi, which is not only responsible for respiratory functions but also for the proper operation of the heart.

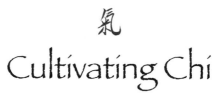

Cultivating Chi

Even though we can name and describe the various types of chi and what they do, chi can never be fully understood simply by thinking about it. Chi only becomes a tangible force when you begin to cultivate it. Cultivate is a particularly appropriate word because, like living things, chi must be nourished and encouraged to develop. And by cultivating chi, we not only come to understand it, we also improve our health.

The Chinese have developed techniques of cultivating chi through exercises called chi kung, which means the practice or art of cultivating the chi. But other cultures have also devised systems of exercises to nurture chi. The first of these systems appeared in the Western world in the form of yoga from India. Certain martial arts arrived at this time, too, including judo and karate, kung fu, and tai chi chuan. Among the last arrivals were the techniques related specifically to chi kung. In the last decade, chi kung practices have become so popular that they have moved out of the traditional confines of the martial arts studios and traditional Chinese medicine and become more mainstream. Today North Americans and Europeans from all walks of life join fellow chi kung-practitioners in Asia in regular daily practice and have learned to appreciate its health benefits.

Chi Kung for Health and Longevity

Although chi kung exercises are often used in connection with the martial arts, traditional healing methods, and some religious practices, they are a discipline unto themselves. In terms of personal health, by learning to cultivate chi, we can prevent disease and even prolong our lives. It is said that chi kung practitioners, who specialize in the art of cultivating personal chi, have lived to the exceedingly old age of one hundred, one hundred-fifty, and even two hundred years or more. In fact, there is a saying that if a Taoist priest, often a chi kung practitioner, dies before the age of one hundred twenty, it is an early death.

Traditional Chinese theory maintains that aging is a process that consumes ever more of the diminishing resources of our bodies, particularly chi. Once the supply is depleted, weakness, illness, and death follow. Fortunately for us, Chinese mystics, philosophers, herbalists, and medical practitioners have discovered a number of ways to supplement our personal store of chi. Their research has yielded a great deal of information and an endless supply of stories.

One such tale recounts the unusual case of Li Ching-Yuen. This famous herbalist and chi kung practitioner was born in 1678, in Chyi Jiang Hsien, in the province of Szechuan. Living most of his life as a recluse in the mountains, he was married 14 times, outliving each of his wives in turn. In 1927, General Yang Sen photographed this man, reputed to be two hundred fifty years of age. Following Li Ching-Yuen's account of his own history, the general later traced the available facts of the case. All indications were that this man had indeed lived for two and a half centuries.

Chi Kung

功氣

Every once in a long while, when walking along a fence bordering a field, you'll notice a single blade of hay protruding from both sides of a fence pole. Only a gust of wind traveling at the right speed and moving in the right direction could provide the precise amount of force to accomplish this feat. Here nature reveals the power of chi in a quietly spectacular way. This power is the force that chi kung practitioners seek to cultivate.

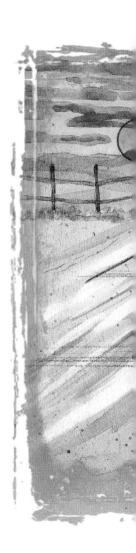

CHAPTER 4

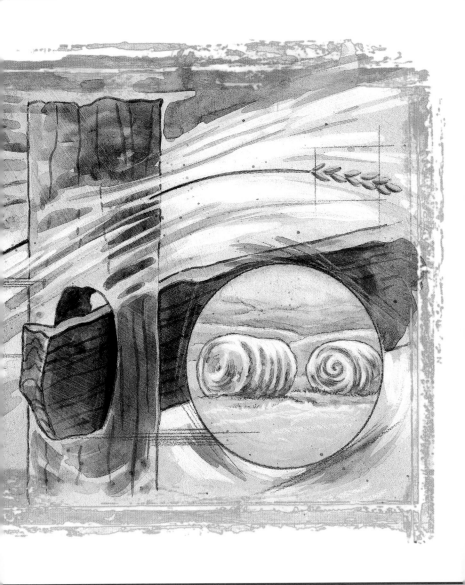

功氣

The Horse Stance

Chi, as we have seen, refers to the living energy in all things. Kung is a term that refers to the achievements of long practice. Together they describe a relationship between someone who cultivates the chi and the discipline they use. Chi kung exercises, then, are used specifically to collect and store chi. The Horse Stance, portrayed in the photograph of the wooden carving (opposite), is known throughout traditional healing and martial arts circles, and it is recognized universally as an extremely beneficial exercise. While there are many variations, the version described here is very basic. Although the posture itself is often found to be difficult and uncomfortable at first, these problems disappear with practice. Usually, a series of special opening and closing movements are used in connection with The Horse, as it is sometimes called. These are designed to promote the movement of chi by opening and closing certain channels in the body, well-known to acupuncturists and other practitioners of traditional medicine. However, benefit can be derived simply by practicing The Horse by itself.

Examine the picture of The Horse Stance. Unfortunately, a wooden carving cannot adequately convey the sense of relaxation a practitioner should have. In a well-executed Horse

Stance, the shoulders and back muscles are completely relaxed throughout the exercise. The feet are placed firmly on the ground about shoulder-width apart. In this form of the stance, the

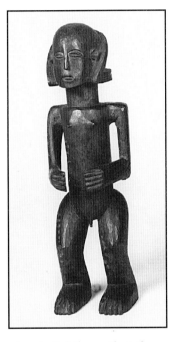

knees are bent slightly so that they are directly above the toes. The arms are raised slowly to waist level with the elbows kept close to the torso, which leans forward slightly. The elbows can be raised or lowered until a comfortable position is found. The exact height of the elbows has an influence on the way chi is absorbed into, and emitted from, the body. The two palms face earthward or sometimes face each other. This is the basic Horse Stance posture.

What is actually happening in the mind of the practitioner is this: The chi is envisioned as moving upward from the ground through the feet, the legs, and past the waist. It flows up along the spinal column, past the shoulders, and into the arms. Then it moves past the elbows and out from the fingers. If the muscles or ligaments are tense in the hips or along the back and shoulders, the chi will be prevented from flowing, and there is no point in continuing the exercise. Practitioners will often step out of the stance until the muscles are once again relaxed. When the chi begins to flow properly, the body begins to rock slowly back and forth, like a supple tree bending in a slight breeze. This is a sign of relaxation. Tense muscles prevent the chi from flowing along the channels. Over time, this stance can be held comfortably for half an hour or more. While standing in The Horse Stance will strengthen the legs, it also has the important function of promoting the flow of chi through the body.

Brought to North America by immigrating Asian chi kung masters and well-traveled Westerners with an interest in the subject, these techniques have remained essentially unchanged during their long migration. The Horse Stance in the photograph is the same basic posture used throughout chi kung history. Even though many variations in the basic stance have developed, the ideas discussed above and demonstrated in the photograph are still in use today.

功氣

Chi Kung: An Ancient Science in Modern Times

Over a period of many hundreds of years, Taoists and others developed many different sets of chi kung exercises. All of them, though, have a common purpose. They attempt to transform the natural energy of chi, found throughout the universe, into a suitable form for use inside the body. This energy can be absorbed from the outside, compressed, stored, and employed in different ways within the body. Some exercises are designed to manipulate chi already inside the body in specialized ways—to heal others, for example, or in the pursuit of enlightenment or in the martial arts. Other exercises move chi through the many acupuncture channels to clear energy blockages. Promoting the free flow of chi to all internal tissues and organs fosters good health. As we will see, these exercises also have many other interesting effects.

Chi Kung Styles

There are many distinct styles of chi kung—more than 2,000 in China alone. Some styles are

Buddhist and others are Taoist. One type of chi kung is comprised largely of standing postures such as The Horse Stance. Practitioners perform the exercises from a stationary position with very few, if any, movements of the feet. These stationary exercises were originally designed to suit the needs of large numbers of monks confined to close quarters in crowded monasteries, temples, and private, nonreligious centers. Such institutions were usually extremely strict in their daily regimen, and the inhabitants often did not have enough exercise to retain good health. Further, their diet was not always sufficient. For this reason, chi kung exercises, sometimes called temple exercises, were developed. These proved doubly useful when monks found themselves imprisoned, not an infrequent occurrence during different periods in Chinese history.

One of the most interesting and highly developed chi kung practices is that of tai chi chuan. Unlike the standing forms, this practice consists of a series of connected movements. Often thought of as a dance, tai chi chuan is actually a moving meditation in which all parts of the body, including the internal organs, are exercised and massaged. While beginners require a small room to practice in, those advanced in the discipline need only a few square feet. In addition to being a chi kung practice, tai chi chuan is also a highly effective martial art. We will study tai chi chuan in some detail in Chapter 6.

功氣

The Origins of Chi Kung

Many chi kung practitioners believe it was a wandering monk who brought the revered art to China. In 475 A.D., Bodhidharma, also known as

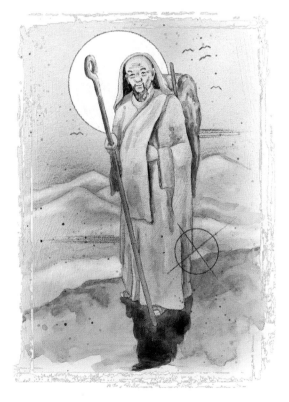

Da Mo, brought not only Buddhist chi kung but also kung fu and an early form of Zen Buddhism, known as Chan, to China from southern India. Buddhist versions of chi kung generally trace their origins to Da Mo, who in later life founded the famous Shaolin temple, located in East China on Mount Sung in Honan Province. Today it serves primarily as a tourist site for vacationers. Other practitioners, however, believe that a form of chi kung originated with Taoist monks many centuries before in China itself and that two distinct forms of the art exist today. Naturally, since two different religions are involved, both schools have distinct ritual traditions, ceremonial observances, and practices for the mind, body, and spirit. Exactly how these practices differ would be the subject for a lengthy book.

Still another closely allied group flourished in Tibet and became the Vajrayana Buddhists. This sect also developed its own special set of chi kung practices. Each of these schools has many similarities not only in chi kung practice but also on key points of doctrine and philosophy, which clearly indicates at least some common founding principles.

Chi Kung and the Cultural Revolution

During the Chinese cultural revolution, however, a pronounced effort was made by the government to purge chi kung and other associated arts of their religious associations. The intent was to "purify" the practices. In the case of chi kung, what survived during this period were techniques that could be used exclusively to promote health. Governmental officials endorsed these exercises and even assisted in formalizing instruction and in promoting chi kung practice among the general population. These sterilized versions of chi kung have little or nothing to say about several of their original purposes, including the notion of the return to Tao and the ideas of immortality and enlightenment. Fortunately, these sacred ideas

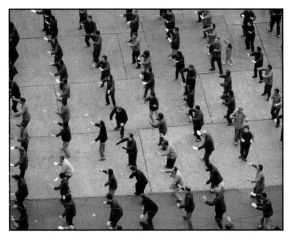

were preserved in secret during these difficult years by dedicated monks and others, often at the peril of losing their lives. Today, they are being reintroduced wherever chi kung is practiced, even, to some extent, in China itself.

The efforts by Chinese officials to purge religion from the face of the earth were especially virulent in Tibet, which China invaded in 1950. Thousands of monasteries, where chi kung, among other disciplines, was traditionally studied and practiced, were completely destroyed. This destruction was a great tragedy for the Tibetan people since monasteries served not only as centers for religious instruction but as centers for education of all types. When these institutions were obliterated, the educated classes were uprooted and the entire history and culture of Tibetan society was in danger of being lost. Fortunately, a great many monks set out to cross the Himalayan mountains, the highest mountains in the world, to escape into Nepal. They brought all that they could carry on their backs, especially their spiritual treasures, including ancients texts passed down through the generations. This harsh pilgrimage cost thousands of lives.

The Study of Animal Behavior: A Living Library of Movement

Constant practice and refinement of chi kung techniques began to yield a number of intriguing results, not the least of which was robust health for the monks confined to the monasteries. From time to time, chi kung practitioners also experienced profound psychological transformations, which led to superior intellectual abilities and even unusual psychic abilities such as telepathy and the ability to see auras. The monks realized that these breakthroughs were related to the chi kung practices themselves. They also realized that the powerful energies they were culti vating could be applied *(continued on page 134)*

HEALTH TIPS FROM ANIMALS

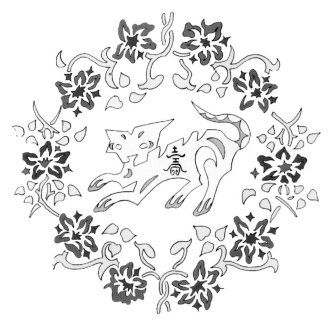

If you have ever watched a cat at rest, you probably noticed that before it moves, it stretches. First it extends its forepaws, completely flexing the spine in a great arch, and then it reverses the stretch. Only then does the cat begin to move. Young, healthy cats perform this exercise after every rest. Known as "Cat Back," it has been adopted as a posture by yoga practitioners. It not only massages the muscles running near the spine, but also promotes the flow of chi to the spinal region, thereby ensuring a fresh supply of life-giving blood to this all-important anatomical structure. The technique is one way cats retain their suppleness and agility well into old age.

THE TAO OF ZEN

The relationship between Taoism and Zen Buddhism has always been very close. It is interesting to note that Bodhidharma's name derives from two root words, bodhi *and* dharma. *Bodhi is a Sanskrit term that refers to enlightenment. It is often coupled with a second term, such as bodhi-tree, the great tree the historical Buddha, Shakyamuni, sat beneath while seeking enlightenment, or Bodhisattva, which indicates a person who is seeking, but has not yet found, enlightenment. The second term, dharma, is another Sanskrit term used to refer to anything "real," that is, anything that transcends the mundane world. It is often used by Buddhists, for example, to indicate the teachings of the historical Buddha after his awakening. It can have as many as ten distinct meanings, including properties (as in characteristics), teachings, events, facts, and reality.*

In many ways, Bodhidharma's teachings are similar to the message of Lao Tsu in his book, The Tao Te Ching. *Even a brief examination of the two systems will reveal a number of parallels. In fact, when Bodhidharma used the word dharma, it was translated by the Chinese as meaning Tao. Aspects of the following passage, paraphrased from Bodhidharma's "The Bloodstream Sermon," could easily be mistaken for the work of a Taoist. It is no wonder the Chinese of the period thought that Chan Buddhism, later to be known as Zen Buddhism in Japan, was simply an Indian version of Taoism.*

The sutras [one of 10,000 sermons presented by the historical Buddha Shakyamuni during his lifetime] *present us with a paradox. They tell us to laugh without laughing, to hear without hearing, and to know without knowing. But what is meant? Move away from language and thought. Move deeper into the true nature of the mind. Doing so, we realize that our worldy experiences enslave us, making us into puppets. What we hear and see, how we feel, and even what we know all conspire to make us react. Only by recognizing emptiness, rather than sensory infomation, as the true nature of the mind, can we escape this vicious circle.*

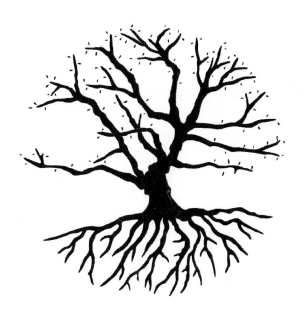

in self defense, a very useful application since in those days traveling monks were easy prey to bands of roving thieves.

By observing animals in their native habitat, the monks discovered exactly how the chi cultivated in their chi kung exercises might be applied in hand-to-hand combat. Due to anatomical peculiarities, such as the long powerful wings of the crane or the extreme flexibility and constricting abilities of the snake, each animal has a unique set of movements that lend themselves well to self-defense and self-preservation in general. The rapierlike beak of the woodpecker, for example, not only pecks deep holes in trees during its search for insects, but serves as a formidable weapon against competitors or enemies. In the water, the snapping turtle is a powerful and graceful swimmer. But on land, it appears to be a a clumsy creature, often hiding deep within its shell. Don't let this subterfuge fool you, however. Its extremely long neck is ready to shoot out of its shell to capture prey at any moment. When it goes fishing, its razor-sharp jaws and vicelike grip make short work of anything that happens to be caught.

Many chi kung exercises are very likely derived from these same kinds of observations. As you might expect, exercises such as The Horse Stance and, in tai chi chuan, Stork Cools Wings, are named after animals and their movements. Some creatures' movements are adopted from real life while others, such as the old favorites, the dragon and the phoenix, are mythical. In terms of self-defense, animal movements were adapted as far as human anatomy would permit. In this way, practitioners learned to imitate the

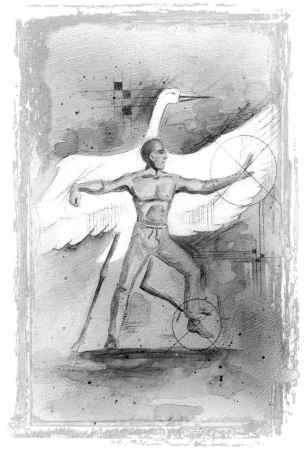

lightening strike of a snake's head, the soft yet powerful blow of a crane's wing, and the raking gouge of the tiger's claw.

功氣

Spiritual Development:
Psychic Powers, Immortality, and Enlightenment

One very practical way to classify chi kung exercises is to separate them into two groups—those related to spiritual concerns and conducted specifically to achieve enlightenment and those related to physical concerns and used to condition the body and to help it resist disease. Some of these latter practices are performed for the benefit of others and are directly related to traditional healing practices, while some are associated with personal, worldly concerns, such as winning a martial arts competition or developing great physical prowess. The most advanced styles of chi kung, such as tai chi chuan, pursue all of these goals at once.

Contemporary chi kung practice is, in a general sense, largely concerned with personal health. But there are many exercises, some still held in confidence, that focus on the development of psychic abilities and even seek to achieve immortality and enlightenment. Some

FIVE DEVA POWERS AND
THE LEAGUE OF THE
IMMORTALS

Certain chi kung masters speak of five extraordinary powers that chi kung practitioners can develop. They are called Deva powers, after powerful supernatural beings. Deva Vision enables remote viewing of events in distant places. This is accomplished with the mind's inner eye, which functions something like a movie screen. Deva Hearing works in a similar way using the inner ear to overhear conversations from great distances. Tell Life is the capacity to disclose previous incarnations of other people. Travel Beyond is the endowment to travel in different dimensions. Other's Heart is the capacity to know another person's innermost thoughts. Legend has it that when a practitioner masters these skills, he or she will enter a fellowship (more of a general distinction than an active group) known as the League of the Immortals, which surpasses the reach of ordinary people.

If these special psychic faculties, or some form of them, really do exist, they may develop as a byproduct of chi kung exercises. So, even if the practitioner's goal is simply to regain lost health or to move energy through the body, these types of extraordinary gifts may also result. Some masters, often from a religious order, specifically warn against consciously setting out to cultivate these powers, however, since their acquisition may lead the practitioner away from what they consider to be the more important goal of enlightenment.

masters often closely guard certain details of their practice, reserving them for their favorite and most trustworthy students. If followed carefully, these practices are reputed to heighten consciousness to superhuman levels (see "Five Deva Powers and the League of the Immortals" on page 137) and dramatically increase the flow of chi in the acupuncture channels of the body. One such exercise, which draws heavily on the forces of nature, is really a type of meditation called Rabbit Salutes the Goddess of Mercy.

Chinese legend has it that the Lady of Compassion, Quan Lin, lives on the moon. Her pet, a rabbit made of jade, stands on the earth saluting her. The jade rabbit, with its red eyes, is well known in the Orient. This meditation gathers energy from the moon. It is performed during the night of the full moon and for each of the three days before and after it. While standing in some place that is very still, watch for the moon to rise above the trees. Cup your hands and raise them to ear level, placing your palms forward. Stand naturally with your knees slightly bent. The meditation is simply to stand quietly, as if in greeting, and watch the moon as it moves through the heavens. Some people feel a breeze blowing through their palms. This is the chi essence of the moon. Only perform the exercise in summer when it is warm. According to traditional Chinese medicine, cold weather can sometimes influence the body in a negative way, particularly when it is in a receptive state such as during the practice of chi kung. This exercise affects your body fluids, which, like the ocean tides, respond to the gravitational pull of the moon. It promotes the flow of the chi in the feminine, or yin, acupuncture channels in the body.

Unlike Rabbit Salutes the Goddess of Mercy, many meditations are performed while seated. Some of these focus on the Du or Governing Channel, which runs along the spine, and attempt to move chi up the spine and through the Baihui point, known as the crown chakra in yogic practice. When the Baihui point is penetrated, a stream of chi flows heavenward through the body. In this way, heaven and earth are symbolically reunited through the free-flowing chi. Those who are successful in this meditation are able to absorb and emit chi simultaneously, a very important ability for those who use chi in healing practice.

Almost unanimously, people who claim to have experienced these awakenings say they have gained insight into the nature of life and existence. By all accounts, it is practically impossible for them to relate the totality of their insights. Many of these fortunate individuals rely on demonstrating, as best they can, their revelations through various art forms such as poetry, painting, and descriptive prose.

Other chi kung practitioners work confidently towards immortality. Some practitioners in this group understand immortality as the development of an imperishable spirit known as *shen*. One indication of the presence of shen is that the practitioner possesses a heightened sense of awareness, an elevated state of mind in which new

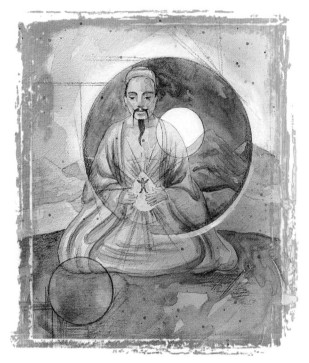

forms of perception are possible. Still other practitioners seek to prolong their lives for unusual lengths of time.

The Secret of the Golden Flower

In 1794, Liu Hua-yang, a monk from the Double Lotus Flower Monastery in Anhui Province in China, consigned an oral teaching to writing. The teachings themselves, later entitled *The Secret of the Golden Flower (T'ai I Chin Hua Tsung Chih)*, originated sometime in the eighth century. It explains in detail some of the theory behind closely guarded chi kung methods for prolonging life. Interestingly, these explanations draw upon both Taoist and Buddhist theory, indicating that a formal exchange of ideas took place between the two movements. These techniques were developed to preserve and supplement the chi already existing in the body. As we have seen in Chapter 3, proper circulation of the chi is believed to restore sick or degenerating tissues and keep them healthy for an indeterminate length of time.

The text makes it clear that the way to longer life, and even to immortality, is through the creation of an eternal spirit body that resides within the physical form. Later, this spirit body separates from the physical body and is born into its own existence. According to Taoist philosophy, such a spirit has to be created individually, earned through painstaking practice and experimentation. As you might imagine, the creation of an immortal spirit body could not possibly be a simple, straightforward process. Even when following elaborate instructions such as those hinted at in *The Secret of the Golden Flower*, because of individual differences, a certain degree of trial and error has always been required to achieve the desired results.

THE SYMBOLISM OF THE GOLDEN FLOWER

The traditional symbol for the Golden Flower is either the lotus or water lily. Its roots grow from a tuber that is firmly planted in mud, submerged beneath the water. This symbolizes the yin force, the chi of the earth, fertile and nurturing, dark and hidden. The roots draw nourishment for the plant from mother earth in her most primal aspect.

In human anatomy, the womb corresponds to the tuber. The roots are like the blood vessels and the invisible psychic channels that nourish the embryo. From this mysterious source, a stem grows, relying on the powerful energies lying latent within the marsh. The stem, which curves and winds its way to the surface, represents both the human spinal column and its associated acupuncture channel known as the Du.

The mission of the plant is to reach the pure, unfiltered sunlight at the surface. The objective of the chi kung practitioner is to reach a higher state of consciousness. Along the plant's stem, which represents the spinal column, run the energy currents. These currents are known to many different cultures. In Indian theory, for example, they are called the Kundalini, or Serpent Power. One form of the practice maintains that these energy currents are actually transmuted sexual energy. It is this energy—this refined chi—that is believed to nourish the mind. Neither the plant nor the practitioner, however, will achieve the mark unless suitable environmental conditions are present.

Once the stem reaches the surface, a single stunning white flower develops. This represents the flowering of the earth energy in the presence of the yang force
of the heavens, represented by sunlight, a symbol of
wisdom and strength. The flower itself represents the
awakened human consciousness. Symbolically, it is
sometimes depicted as a lotus flower in full bloom

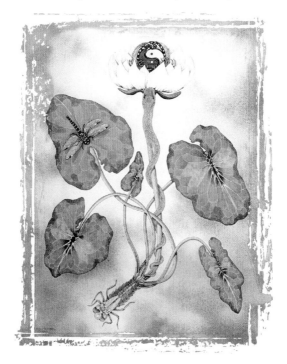

above the head. The energies that bring it to life flow
through the Baihui acupoint on the crown of the head.

In Taoist tradition, the flowering of consciousness
is associated with immortality since it not only can
lead to superior mental skills but also, in many cases,
to superb physical health as well.

功氣
The Problem of Authenticity

In modern times, chi kung instructions are very precise, and students inevitably require an experienced teacher to teach them correctly. Otherwise, they will likely become lost and confused. But chi kung practice was not always so elaborate. How could it be? Today, we have the benefit of centuries of experience, much of which has been recorded and incorporated into the chi kung forms themselves.

Today, after 2,000 years or so of continuous development, a great number of chi kung systems use a highly structured, even rigorous, training curriculum. Still, the basic ideas of the ancients remain at the heart of chi kung practice, though the curriculum now incorporates the discoveries of generations of practitioners. This means that not only the original postures and applications but also their derivations and some that are entirely new must also be mastered. The only way to transmit this enormous collection of findings properly is through systematic training. With each successive generation of students, variations in the exercises, known as forms, have been developed. Naturally, over the course of centuries, the original forms were obscured until very few, if any, can be said to be identical to the original exercises.

Claiming a Lineage

Fortunately, there are several ways to verify whether any particular practice is indeed genuinely related to the original instructions. All

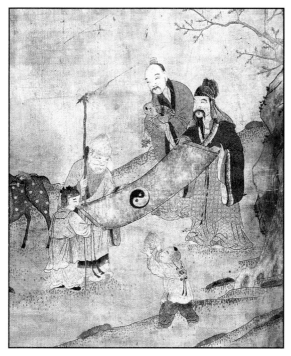

Asian teachings, whether they are religious, martial, or healing in nature, claim a lineage, or membership in a particular school. Even today, lineage is a source of great pride for practitioners, and internecine rivalry is common. The importance of one's lineage is determined by the abilities and

fame of its members, past and present. To be able to claim a lineage is akin to holding a passport into exclusive societies, similar to the social advantages possessed by members of a privileged caste, that is totally inaccessible to average citizens. In fact, highly respected chi kung practitioners in Asia are often revered as gods with magical powers, and their names are prefixed with the title "Divinity."

Another way to verify an authentic chi kung practice is by its results. If the method is successful and if well-known practitioners verify that it can accomplish what it claims, such as better health, the development of unusual abilities, and so on, the practice will be accepted. If not, its chances for survival are greatly diminished.

A final way to verify a system is to compare its central ideas with those of the formal doctrines. In Taoist thought, these texts include notable works from many disciplines such as the *I Ching* (philosophy), the *Tao Te Ching* (philosophy), *The Inner Classic of the Yellow Emperor* (medicine), *The Secret of the Golden Flower* (mysticism), and the eight tai chi chuan classics themselves (discussed in Chapter 6).

These texts and others like them contain the seminal ideas that are reflected in all authentic schools. While allowing for some departure and modification, the core principles taught by any particular instructor will generally adhere to the standards set in these texts. After all, the classics

GOPI KRISHNA AND THE
FLOWERING OF
CONSCIOUSNESS

The following account, by Gopi Krishna, describes his own experience when the chi, or prana as it is called in India, began to circulate throughout his body. At the time of his awakening, he was a clerk with the Department of Education in Kashmir, a province in northern India.

"Suddenly," he began, "with a roar like that of a waterfall, I felt a stream of liquid light entering my brain through the spinal cord. The illumination grew brighter and brighter, the roaring louder, I experienced a rocking sensation and then felt myself slipping outside of my body, entirely enveloped in a halo of light. I was no longer myself, but instead was a vast circle of consciousness in which the body was but a point, bathed in light and in a state of exaltation and happiness impossible to describe."

When these states of being become permanent and the chi flows freely through all of the channels in the body, legend has it that the chi kung practitioner joins the League of the Immortals. At this point they acquire the Deva powers and are capable of superhuman feats. According to tradition, immortals do not seem to die, they simply join the gods and populate the heavenly kingdom. Chinese legends are replete with stories of the immortals.

have formed the basis for discussion and commentary throughout history. Because they have endured, they are the final standard by which all practices are measured.

功氣

The Importance of Intention in Chi Kung

Not everyone who follows the techniques will achieve what they intend. Some masters and many references in both Taoist and Buddhist texts issue clear warnings: Those who squander or abuse their energies in the pursuit of worldly pleasures and those who are simply evil will be unable to control the forces they unleash. The reason is this: Only if the mind is pure will the chi be able to circulate upward to illuminate it, thereby inducing enlightenment and stimulating the creative forces associated with heaven. If the mind is impure—that is, focused on unwholesome thoughts or ambitions—the chi will be attracted to and migrate to equally coarse energies associated with the lower realms of existence.

In Taoist folklore, fox spirits are said to inhabit these lower realms. Foxes, as well as people, are believed to be able to cultivate the elixir of life, which leads to the creation of a spirit body. As a result, foxes are occasionally thought to move up the evolutionary totem pole and reincarnate in human form. But if we, who are already human, abuse the energies created in our efforts to form a spirit body, then we may descend into the lower realms and find ourselves reincarnated as a fox spirit. There, for perhaps a thousand years or more, we will roam free and happy in mountains under the light of sun and moon and stars. But, at last, we will be reborn into this same world, a world of strife and suffering.

功氣

The Backward Flowing Method

As we have seen in Chapter 3, parents impart a limited amount of prenatal chi to their children at birth. This finite quantity suggests its importance to our health and well-being and that it is vital to conserve and supplement it. The monks focused their attention on developing special chi kung techniques that would redirect chi along the energy channels we know as acupuncture meridians. These pathways often become clogged in adult life, so these chi kung exercises help to restore the chi to a natural and efficient flow through the body.

Essentially, the many chi kung techniques developed by the monks are designed "to reverse the flow of chi" so that the mind no longer needlessly directs it to perform the menial tasks of the exterior world. While we naturally require chi simply to exist, chi kung practice teaches us not only to supplement the supply in our bodies, but to be more efficient in its use. Typically, we simply give up certain habits that we recognize as interfering with our progress. We also learn to meditate and to discipline ourselves so that our attention does not wander and our energies are not dissipated while we perform a task.

Transmutation of Sexual Energy

But the phrase "reversing the flow" has another meaning, more complex than the general description offered above. It refers to a complex, multistage chi kung practice that, according to Taoist methods, involves the transmutation of sexual, or "seed," energy. Metaphorically speaking, the "seed" energy represents the creative potential that is latent within our bodies. We can express this potential in either of two ways. We can follow our biological instincts and mate and have children. Or, we can sublimate these primal impulses, redirect them, and express them as artistic creations, in the martial arts, in healing techniques, or in the pursuit of enlightenment. How it might be possible to chemically alter physical substances in the body has been the subject of much debate and study over the centuries. The results of these efforts are the chi kung techniques we use today.

Through the practice of chi kung, the powerful reproductive instinct can be controlled. At this point, it becomes possible to awaken special processes that lie latent in the body and ultimately to induce the flowering of consciousness. The first of these is the attempt to transmute the seminal energy from a physical substance directed toward the reproductive activities to form chi that can be used within the body. This process of seed energy conversion is a fundamental aspect of Taoist alchemy. The second process is the attempt to direct the chi up the spine through a number of acupoints to the brain. The third process is the attempt to nourish and sustain the shen, or spirit, which is believed to reside in the area of the forehead located between the eyes. When the spirit is sufficiently developed (some say it typically takes three years), it can be used in the pursuit of the final goal of enlightenment.

Typically, breathing exercises coupled with meditation are used to bring about these effects. Once perfected, the method leads to the flowering or expansion of consciousness, hence the phrase "golden flower," described earlier in this chapter. The idea of sublimating sexual energy was elaborated upon by Sigmund Freud, the father of psychoanalysis, and used as a central concept in psychoanalytic theory.

功氣

The Greater and Lesser Circulation

Taoist chi kung techniques focus on balancing and strengthening the energies in the body. Practitioners noticed that when chi flows abundantly, smoothly, and correctly through all the channels in the body, a substance called shen, an imperishable spirit, develops naturally. They also noticed that in our daily lives most of us tend to expend chi in futile, even self-destructive ways. The general movements with which we perform our daily activities, for example, are often exaggerated or executed without regard to maximum efficiency. This results in a needless loss of valuable chi and tends to retard the development of shen. Further, many of us have little regard for our posture. As a consequence, the internal organs of the body become cramped and the acupuncture channels become blocked. We also senselessly dissipate chi by indulging ourselves excessively when eating, drinking, or engaging in any other common activity. Two techniques central to Taoist chi kung, known as the Greater and Lesser Circulation, are commonly used to restore chi to different parts of our body.

When the chi flows smoothly without interruption through the two most central channels, the Du or Governing Channel, which runs up the spinal column, and the Ren or Conception Channel, which follows a line along the center of the front of the body, the chi kung practitioner has accomplished a feat known as the Lesser Circulation. When chi flows without interruption throughout all twelve major channels in the body, as well as the Du and the Ren, another major attainment, The Greater Circulation, has been accomplished. Movement of chi in these two orbits is considered in some schools to be a precursor to the further strengthening and control of the chi.

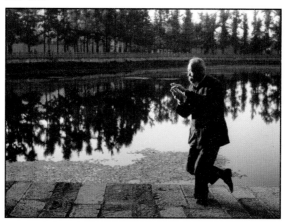

Accounts of these states typically describe an experience of heightened awareness and elevated consciousness. Often referred to as awakenings because of the special psychological and even mystical insights that accompany them, these states have a profound impact on those who experience them. It is invariably accompanied by a sense of the eternal and an absolute certainty that each of us is now and always has been an integral part of the endless interplay of cosmic forces. To know these things with an incontestable certainty is to know something about immortality.

功氣

Healing Applications

Certain versions of chi kung have been developed exclusively for use in healing applications. Typically, these methods focus specifically on strengthening the chi and on learning to emit it to heal others. Healing chi kung techniques are taught and practiced openly throughout much of the modern world, including China where they are officially endorsed. In fact, chi kung healers can be found in private practice in any large city in North America or Europe. In Asia they are often associated with hospitals.

The New World Press, located in Bejing, reported as early as 1984 that Shanghai No. 8 People's Hospital has been using a form of chi kung to induce anesthesia in patients about to have surgery. In these situations, chi kung is sometimes used to supplement drugs and sometimes as an anesthetic by itself. The report also noted that Chinese nuclear scientists were conducting experiments on chi in an attempt to find out how it works. They discovered that it was a type of "low frequency modulated infrared radiation" that can be emitted by certain individuals.

There are many other healing applications of chi as well. All chi kung practitioners learn to collect universal chi by absorbing it through chi gates and storing it in their bodies. But the many chi kung practitioners who also learn to emit chi are reputedly able to transmit it without actually touching the other person. Known as *wei chi,* or out-flowing chi, this form of chi can be projected for a distance of 16 feet. For healing purposes, though, the distance between practitioner and subject is generally between one and three feet. Practitioners who are able to emit chi in this way are held in high regard in official circles, and many are invited to annual conferences where, among other things, they treat senior government officials.

Over time, certain chi kung practitioners claim to have developed a sixth sense that enables them to visually scan the internal organs and tissues of their clients for weakness and illnesses. They have learned to associate the different colors they see with different diseases. This ability helps the chi kung master to identify illness and pathogenic conditions. These auras are described as a light radiating outward from the diseased parts of the body. Typically, blue lights are associated with a deficiency of yang or hot chi and red lights are associated with a deficiency of yin or cold chi. Green is often associated with

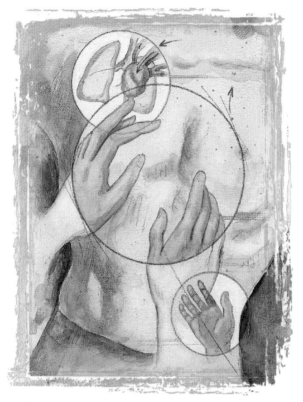

infection or poison and yellow or brown with bruises and sprains. Black indicates dead tissue and an absence of chi altogether.

In a typical chi kung healing session, the patient will lie fully clothed on a treatment table. The chi kung practitioner may ask the client a number of health-related questions or may simply begin to emanate wei chi. According to the theory, the wei chi strengthens the patient's personal chi to the point at which it becomes visible to the practitioner. This kind of X-ray vision can be regarded as an example of a Deva power. At this point, the practitioner makes an assessment as to which parts of the body are unhealthy, which organs are affected, which acupuncture channels are associated with the organs, which prominent acupuncture points lie on those channels, and which type of chi kung treatment should be used.

Other practitioners see nothing unusual at all. They rely instead on a highly refined sense that develops around the hands. These practitioners typically feel one of a number of sensations radiating upward from the body. The hands need not even touch the client but simply feel vibrations through the air. In this way, the chi kung practitioner can isolate problem areas in the body. There are well over a dozen different qualities of chi that are recognized in medical chi kung. Chinese pulse-reading doctors, famous throughout the world for their diagnostic abilities, are able to sense these same qualities by feeling the many variations in the pulse of their clients.

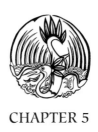

CHAPTER 5

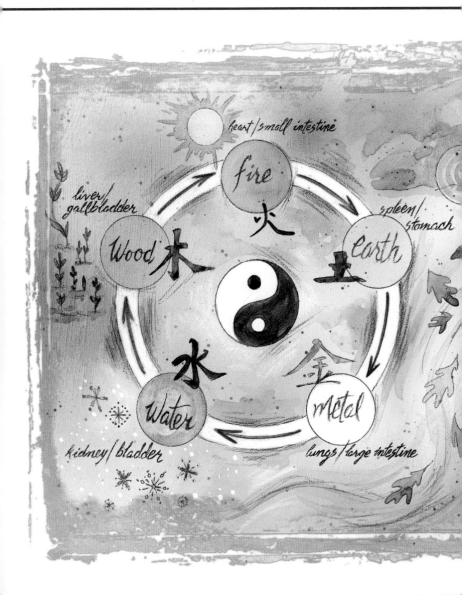

Traditional Chinese Medicine

針灸

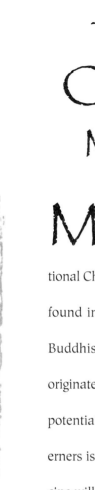

Much of the theory behind traditional Chinese medicine is based on ideas found in the *I Ching* and in Taoist and Buddhist philosophy. Since these ideas originate in a nonWestern worldview, the potential for misunderstanding by Westerners is great. Traditional Chinese medicine will be easier to understand, then, if its ideas are not interpreted too literally. Instead, recall the mythology and imagery in the ancient writings, and seek the spirit of traditional Chinese medicine there.

針灸

Chinese Healing

After looking at some of the principal ideas in traditional Eastern philosophy, it is easy to discern that a medical system based on those ideas has little in common with modern Western medicine. This does not mean that the Eastern system has no value. On the contrary, it suggests that modern Western medicine may have overlooked or forgotten very viable means of detecting, diagnosing, and treating illness. Eastern techniques rely on the fundamental concepts discussed earlier in the book: the concepts of yin and yang, of balancing those two energies, and of the unity of human life and nature.

Since traditional Chinese medicine is rooted in Chinese philosophy, to understand its methods we must learn to understand health and the human body in a new way. Health, according to traditional Chinese medicine, is a reflection of our relationship to our environment. The human body is considered to be a microcosmic reflection of the greater universe, and the relationship between the individual and the surrounding world is always of paramount importance. What we eat, say, do, and think, who we associate with, and even our occupations all affect our health.

This idea is reflected in a number of oriental arts besides medicine, including feng shui, the

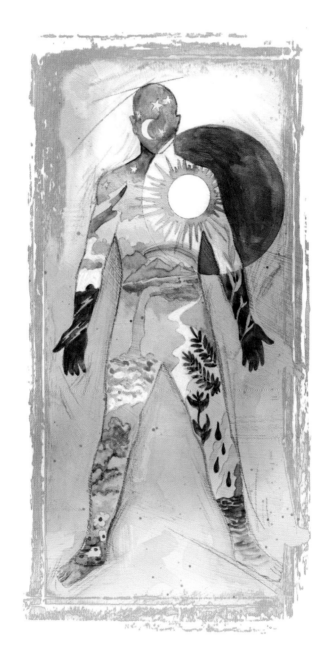

WISDOM OF TAI CHI

161

ancient art of positioning one's home and work spaces in a way that is harmonious with the environment. According to feng shui theory, buildings, even rooms, are influenced by natural forces. When a structure is designed in harmony with those forces, they will support the structure and its occupants. In the same way, good health dictates that our personal relationship with the surrounding world must always be complementary. So, when we become ill, the Chinese physician first seeks an imbalance within the patient and then looks for a cause in the external environment.

In terms of medical practice, a Western allopathic physician might simply treat the diseased organ with a drug or perhaps with surgery. A traditional Chinese medical practitioner, though, treats the patient as a whole, not just the affliction, and attempts to restore harmony within the patient and between the patient and the surrounding world. Ultimately, a balance in this relationship leads to a balancing of yin and yang energies in the body and, as a consequence, restoration of health and vitality. Techniques such as massage, chi kung, acupuncture, moxibustion, herbal formulas, dietary and lifestyle changes, and exercise therapy are all used in this effort.

In traditional practice, it is important to find the root of the disease, the source of the imbalance. It is not sufficient simply to say that the cause of a particular illness is a viral infection, for example. A traditional practitioner must trace the origins of the disease even further, to be able to explain exactly why the virus was able to gain access to the body in the first place. Only then, when the root is discovered, can the imbalance be reversed.

針灸

The Methods of Diagnosis

In traditional Chinese medicine, then, illness is understood as the consequence of disharmony in the body's energy system. In terms of diagnosis, this idea of balance provides a framework for a simple, yet immensely practical diagnostic tool known as the four examinations. The techniques are organized into four groups.

The Four Examinations

The inspection, known less formally as "the looking exam," involves studying the patient's external appearance. The practitioner studies the patient's general vitality; facial coloration; appearance, including posture and movements; the eyes, nose, ears, gums, mouth, and throat; and the tongue. The study of the tongue provides the physician with especially important diagnostic information. Heart conditions, for instance, are suggested by a crack running down the center of the tongue. Coatings on the tongue, called "moss," are related to the digestive system, and different colored coatings, such as green, blue, yellow, and gray, each indicate a specific medical problem.

Auscultation and olfaction are technical terms that refer to listening and smelling. In this exam, the physician listens to the timbre of the voice during speech and to respiratory characteristics exhibited during breathing and coughing. Particular types of body odors are also noted.

The interrogation is an inquiry by the physician into the patient's medical history and lifestyle. The physician will note the presence or absence of chills, fevers, perspiration, appetites, thirsts, changes in elimination patterns, characteristics of stool and urine, specific pains, sleeping patterns, and common ailments such as headaches.

Palpation means to examine through the sense of touch. Using a highly discriminating sense of touch, the traditional Chinese medical practitioner searches for imbalances of yin or yang energy within the different organs and mechanisms of the body. This exam includes touching the upper and lower abdomen, the hands, the feet, and the acupuncture points. But the emphasis in this exam is on the pulse of the radial artery of both wrists. Each of the wrists is associated with a different grouping of organs. The heart, liver, and one kidney are found on the left side, and the lungs, spleen, and other kidney

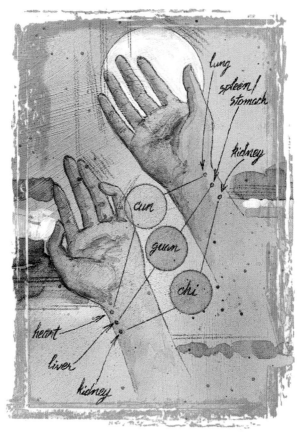

are associated with the right. Using this technique, the physician reads as many as 30 different types of pulse, each indicating a different condition in the body. A pulse, for example, can be superficial or deep, slow or rapid, deficient or excessive, rolling or hesitant, and so on. Typically, a disease will create a pulse that exhibits two or more of these characteristics. Determining its nature, then, can be an involved and difficult process.

The Differentiation of Syndromes

Each of the four types of observation provides the physician with specific information about the patient's health. Patterns and relationships between the organs and mechanisms of the body are then sought out by using this information in conjunction with a special classification system known as the Differentiation of Syndromes. This system provides a matrix that enables the physician to organize information relating to the patient in progressively finer degrees. Correct correlation of the patient's symptoms with the appropriate syndromes is the key to successful diagnosis. There are four main systems of classifying syndromes: the eight principles, the theory of chi and blood, the acupuncture channels, and the theory of zang-fu organs.

We have seen how the blood and the chi are related to one another and how they exist co-dependently in the body. The Chinese system of acupuncture channels, which we will discuss in more detail later in this chapter, is an elaborate system of channels through which the chi can flow to every part of the body. It works in much the same way as the circulatory system does for moving blood through the body. The theory of the zang-fu organs and the eight principles are two concepts that we have not yet mentioned. Some knowledge of both ideas, though, is basic to understanding traditional Chinese medicine.

Zang-fu is a classification system for the internal organs that is fundamental to traditional Chinese medicine. Chinese medicine organizes the organs into three categories, the solid yin (or zang) organs, which include the lungs, heart, spleen, liver, and kidney; the hollow yang (or fu) organs, which include the small and large intestines, gallbladder, bladder, stomach, and "triple warmer"—a special term that refers to the working relationship between several organs, rather than to a specific organ itself; and the "extra fu," a group of less important organs in terms of process, which include the brain, uterus, marrow, bone, blood vessels, and gallbladder. (The gallbladder is considered both a fu and an extra-fu organ.) These three organ systems work together to keep the body healthy.

The eight principles is a system of diagnosis according to eight categories, or characteristics, of illness. The principles are organized into four groups of complementary opposites: yin and yang, interior and exterior, cold and hot, deficiency and excess. Yin and yang, however, is the primary category in this system; the other three are actually subcategories. Disharmonies revealed by this system of diagnosis are then appropriately treated.

針灸
Five Element Theory

Like the yin-yang theory, the Five Element Theory is a system of classifying not just objects but processes and the forces of nature. In traditional Chinese medicine, it is another important evaluative tool and is used in conjunction with the methods and systems previously discussed. While the yin-yang theory sought to explain all interactions as two fundamental energies, the theory of the five elements defines the natural world in terms of five fundamental substances, wood, fire, earth, metal, and water. These elements, found in varying degrees in all things, can either work together harmoniously or be out of balance and in opposition to one another. Since the human body is a part of nature, each of its individual components, the various tissues and organs, can be related to one of the five elements. If an organ, for example, is not functioning properly, it is studied in relation to its element and also in terms of how that element should behave when functioning normally.

Each element possesses a distinguishing characteristic that represents a natural activity. The inherent disposition of wood, for example, is to grow, while that of earth is to create and nour-

TABLE OF THE FIVE ELEMENTS AND THEIR CORRESPONDENCES

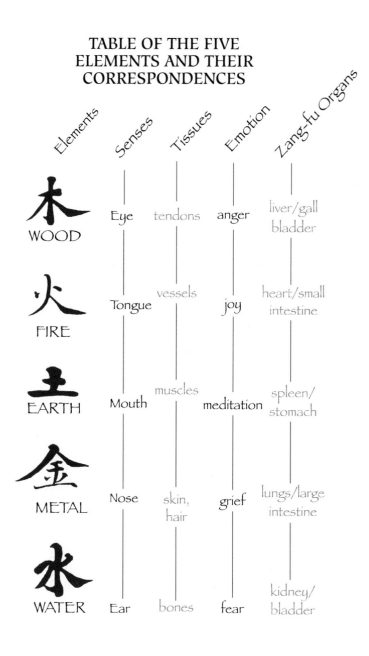

Elements	Senses	Tissues	Emotion	Zang-fu Organs
木 WOOD	Eye	tendons	anger	liver/gall bladder
火 FIRE	Tongue	vessels	joy	heart/small intestine
土 EARTH	Mouth	muscles	meditation	spleen/stomach
金 METAL	Nose	skin, hair	grief	lungs/large intestine
水 WATER	Ear	bones	fear	kidney/bladder

CHANNELING THE CHI

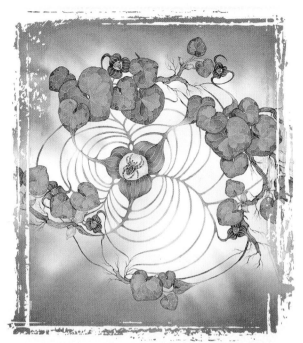

If we could actually witness the inner processes of plant life, we would know that the roots of the wild ginger cover the forest floor, much like a spider's web. The roots spread in an expansive array, carpeting the moist shady ground, drawing up nutrients and precious water. They seem to work collectively, uniting many separate plants. In this sense, the vast network of roots acts much like the elaborate system of acupuncture channels that run throughout the human body, enabling the life-supporting chi to move to all tissues without restriction.

ish; that of fire is to heat and rise up, while that of water is to chill and flow downward; and that of metal is clarity. All five elements support a relationship with one another and many natural processes. The seasons, colors, tastes, emotions, and certain musical notes have all been classified according to the five elements.

The Five Elements and the Process of Change

In the West we tend to rely on fact and empirical evidence. But the Chinese theory of the elements deals with the material world only in a secondary and indirect way. The elements are more than just materials found in the world. They are abstract representations, descriptions of concepts that enable us to see certain patterns of behavior. Essentially, the Five Element Theory defines a set of relationships created during the process of change. The elements themselves represent conditions as they are at their most stable point, just before they actually begin to change.

A helpful way to understand these relationships is to look at how the five elements correspond to the seasons of the year. Wood corresponds to spring, and it is the element associated with youth and growth. Fire corresponds to summer and describes conditions that have reached a peak of activity and are about to rest. Earth signifies a state of balance, or in a sense, a condition between changes, and corresponds to Indian summer.

Metal is related to autumn and represents conditions in a state of decline. Water is related to winter, a condition in which activity is in its deepest state of rest, just about to change direction and begin a new cycle. In this example, it is easy to see a cycle in which spring represents the budding of activity. From that point in the cycle, the activity increases in intensity until it reaches its zenith, and then gradually begins to decline until it reaches a complete state of rest during winter.

This example of the seasons helps us recognize the general manner in which the elements, in the form of the seasons, can interact. Although the seasonal pattern of interaction is linear, with the cycle progressing from wood through fire, earth, metal, and water, the five elements can interact in non-sequential ways. As well as having a relationship with fire, for example, wood, also has a direct relationship with earth and with metal. As we shall see in the next chapter on tai chi chuan, the implications of these relationships have significant consequences.

The five element cycle is reflected in different examples throughout the natural world. The seeds of plants, for example, germinate during the spring. In summer, they grow and develop. By late summer, these plants mature. By autumn, the seeds have fully developed and are scattered. Soon the mother plant will die, the leaves, stalks, and stems providing nourishment, in the form of compost, for the earth itself. Winter is a time for this plant material to begin the process of decomposition, to be assimilated, a time of rest and replenishment for the soil and of preparation for the forthcoming season. Such is the cycle of life: rest, rebirth, youth, maturity, and death. This larger framework, in which all living entities flourish for a time and then recede, has been called the web of life by poets and philosophers. And so, as we move through this web of life, we find our lives, like those of the plants, in a constant state of change.

In some respects, the Five Element Theory can be thought of as an extension of the yin-yang theory and, in fact, the two methodologies are usually closely associated. Both theories are very ancient, and although their exact beginnings are lost, historians have traced the partnership of these two theories through vast eras of time. In the discussion of the yin and the yang, these two primary forces, either negative or positive in character, initially encourage growth and development and later restrict it.

These same two forces can be seen at work within each of the stages of the five element cycle. In the example of wood, we noted that its season was spring. Early spring is a period when the earth is just released from the grip of winter and so is a cold period, yin in character. As spring moves into early summer, the heat from the sun intensifies, and its yin character gradually transforms into yang. This same progression can be seen in different forms from the beginning to the end of the year.

In traditional Chinese medicine, physicians who use the Five Element Theory recognize that the system does tend to oversimplify conditions as they appear in clinical situations. But they also realize that, to a considerable extent, it can be useful in certain diagnostic and prescriptive capacities, largely because it expands the scope of the yin and yang theory. By assigning the different organs to separate elements, for example, the physician has extended the descriptive matrix, making it more comprehensive.

When both theories are combined, it is possible for us to view the human body in a way that more properly reflects its true character, as an organism whose health is directly dependent on the proper coordination and flow of energy between a vast number of interrelated and interdependent parts. Further, the flow of energy considered is not restricted to the processes of the body itself, but extends outside of it, to the exterior world.

In this way, we can think of ourselves as a microcosm, a miniature reflection of the larger processes currently working in the surrounding environment. This thought leads us to the realization that whatever is good for the world around us is also good for human beings—a surprisingly current point of view. As you might expect, the reverse is also true.

針灸
The Theory Behind Acupuncture Therapy

The theories of yin and yang and the five elements offer a general philosophical framework that helps the physician interpret information gathered during the four examinations. The two theories work together, and even though they originated in antiquity, they still provide the basic matrix for clinical practice in traditional Chinese medicine.

Once a diagnosis has been made, the physician has a number of prescriptive tools available, including suggestions for changes in lifestyle, herbal supplements and dietary changes, the use of acupuncture, and the use of moxibustion—the application of burning herbs and heat to injured areas. But to a Westerner, traditional Chinese medicine is most closely associated with acupuncture, the process of inserting hair-fine needles into specific acupoints on the body. Although this technique is not the traditional Chinese medical practitioner's only therapeutic tool, it certainly is one of the most familiar. The basic theory behind its practice is not difficult to understand: Chi must flow smoothly and without interruption throughout the body. When its flow is obstructed, it stagnates, causing disease. Excess or insufficient chi will also adversely affect the body and cause health problems.

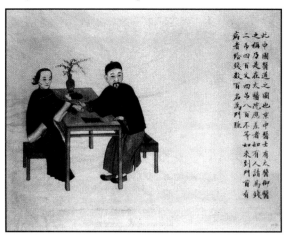

Acupuncture theory has been heavily influenced by the principle of yin and yang. As mentioned in the discussion of zang-fu, each organ is assigned to one of these qualities. The six yang organs begin the process of assimilating food into the body and removing wastes. This is understood as the active function. The yin organs use the food, now partially broken down, to create and manage the fundamental substances themselves: chi, shen, blood, and other body fluids. The nurturing function is clearly visible here. The six extra-fu organs work in a manner similar to the yin organs, but they look like the yang organs.

THE MEANING OF
ACUPOINT NAMES

The traditional acupuncture system organizes acupoints into six categories, each of which describes certain qualities or features. Names of the points were assigned according to the following groupings: water; plants, animals, or instruments; anatomy; astronomy; therapeutic property; or architectural features. The Shaoze point (Small Intestine number one; also Shao-Tze, Shao Ze), for example, translates as Young or Lesser Marsh. Here the chi cools and moistens, creating a marsh-like effect, so this particular reference is very apt. Another reference to water is Jiquan, (Heart number one; also Chi-Ch'uan, Ji Quan), meaning Summit's Spring. This is a reference to the manner in which the chi bubbles to the surface from its underground source deeper in the body. Qiuxu (Gallbladder number 40; also Ch'iu-Hsu, Qiu Xu), is an anatomical reference to the mound on the ankle bone. While the point itself has therapeutic applications, the name is used simply as a marker in the anatomical landscape. The Shenmen point (Heart number seven; also Shen-Men, Shen Men) means Spiritual Gate, an architectural reference that analogously describes the way in which the human spirit, known as shen, may be favorably influenced by manipulation of this point. Many of the traditional acupoint names are still well-known and widely used today.

ACUPUNCTURE: NOT JUST A CHINESE ART

Many countries have used acupuncture as a primary medical treatment, including Tibet, Korea, and Japan. Each of these countries has developed its own system, with its own special variations. Traditional Tibetan doctors, for example, acknowledge substantially more channels than the Chinese—84,000 to be exact—that also carry either blood, chi, or both. All traditions, however, agree on the fundamental ideas behind the system of channels that travel throughout the body. While there are regional and disciplinary differences in names, functions, locations of points, and methods of treatment, there are some features that they all agree upon. One such commonality is that all of these disciplines work to transform internal energies.

Although the exact point locations do not always correspond among these different acupuncture systems, some of them do, and the names and functions of these are often universally known. Practitioners of many different disciplines, such as yoga, Zen, Tibetan Buddhism, and tai chi chuan are familiar with them. The transcultural recognition of these acupoints is due to their importance in moving energy through the body.

針灸

Acupuncture Channels and Acupoints

To understand how acupuncture works, imagine a complex network of very fine channels running throughout the body. These channels carry chi, the life energy, to every cell. Chi flows along these routes in much the same way blood flows through the blood vessels or lymph moves through the lymphatic system.

There are twelve regular channels, fifteen collateral channels, twelve divergent channels, and eight extra channels. Together these channels circulate the chi throughout the entire body. Where one channel ends, the next begins. Each channel travels widely throughout the body, passing through one or more organs. Some of these channels, or parts of them, pass close to the surface of the skin. At periodic intervals along the channels are points at which the chi is readily accessible. Known as acupoints, these places provide access to the chi within a particular channel. Practitioners can influence the activity of the chi within the channel by using acupuncture needles to stimulate it through these acupoints. Some acupoints are of more importance than others, since greater

WORLD HEALTH ORGANIZATION ENDORSES ACUPUNCTURE

The World Health Organization (WHO) is an international association of 190 countries with headquarters in Geneva, Switzerland. Traditional medicine is one of its many interests, since the organization recognizes that much of the world depends upon indigenous medicine. For the last 20 years, WHO has sponsored research into this field and has attempted to determine which traditional medical procedures are effective and which are not. The use of acupuncture has been supported by WHO since the 1970s.

Of the 25 centers for traditional medicine currently collaborating with WHO, seven are conducting research into acupuncture.

According to the WHO report, WHO's Policy and Activities on Traditional Medicine, *there are some 10,000 acupuncture specialists and more than 100,000 Chinese traditional medical doctors practicing acupuncture in China. According to a survey of acupuncture-moxibustion in Europe, in 1990 the total number of acupuncturists had reached 88,000; 62,000 of them were medical doctors. The number of acupuncture users was estimated at 20 million.*

quantities of chi are present at or near these locations. As a result of this accumulation, it is often practical to influence the workings of the body by manipulating the chi at these locations. These special points are commonly known as chi gates.

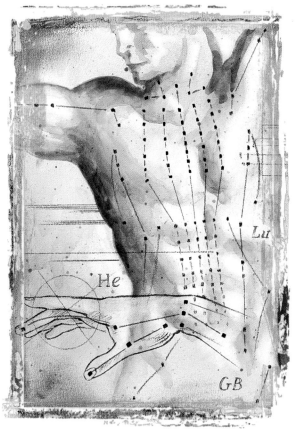

When the acupuncturist believes an organ is weak or diseased, he or she stimulates corresponding points on the relevant channel to restore proper functioning. The chi may be stagnant or there may be excesses or deficiencies of it, all of which can be corrected through acupuncture. More than four hundred points have been charted, most of them located where chi runs near the surface of the body. Since the points vary in depth beneath the surface of the skin, acupuncturists must also know how deeply to penetrate. If the needle is inserted too deeply, it can cause tissue or organ damage.

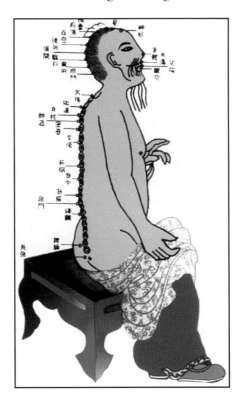

Acupuncture points are classified by number system related to each specific channel. Each channel has a different number of points, and there is a mutually supportive relationship among the channels themselves. As far as the regular channels are concerned, this relationship is sequential; where one channel ends, the next begins. The pathway of the Heart Channel, for example, ends at point number nine, located on the bottom inside edge of the little fingernail. Close to this, on the outside edge of the same nail, the Small Intestine Channel begins. The first point on this channel begins as point number one. For the acupuncturist, the number system is a very convenient way of tracing the path of chi as it moves through the body and of locating the specific points themselves.

In clinical practice, the system of acupoints works in the following way. The Large Intestine Channel, for example, begins on the outside edge of the index finger. It travels up the outside of the arm, to the back of the shoulder and neck. Then it returns to the front of the body and moves up the neck and then across the jaw and mouth to the nostrils. Since this part of the channel runs close to the surface, it is accessible, and there are a number of acupoints along it. Another branch of the channel, however, is inaccessible since it runs deeply inside the body, roughly from the scapula to the large intestine itself. A practitioner may wish to influence the movement of chi in the large intestines to correct a problem such as dysentery or constipation, *(continued on page 186)*

THE HISTORY OF
ACUPUNCTURE

In China, the first ideas about medicine were gathered together at about the same time as the theory of yin and yang began to develop, during what is known as the Clan Period. This era began 100,000 years ago in the prehistoric period of Chinese civilization and is divided into two halves, known as the Old Stone Age and the New Stone Age. In these earliest times, medical knowledge was limited to basic skills such as dietary supplements, lancing and scraping infections, massage, herbal lore, and simple bone setting. Chinese scholars believe that it was in the New Stone Age, approximately 8000 to 2000 B.C., that the science of acupuncture actually began. During this time, ongoing improvements in stone shaping techniques made it possible to manufacture the precise tools required.

The legendary Yellow Emperor, Huang Di, (2690–2590 B.C.), is often credited with the creation of the first acupuncture needles and with developing techniques to use them. Renowned as a great benefactor of the people, he reportedly wrote The Yellow Emperor's Classic of Internal Medicine.

During this period, acupuncture needles were not the sharp, delicate tools we know today. In fact, the needles were made from stone. Known as "Bian Shyr," the needles of the time came in a num-

ber of different shapes and sizes. Some even looked remarkably like arrowheads. Typically, the stones were used to lance an infection, to scrape an abscessed wound, or even to assist in bloodletting procedures. Five hundred years later, a technique known as moxibustion was introduced to work together with or independently from acupuncture.

Later discoveries from the Shang Dynasty (1776–1122 B.C.) demonstrated that thoughtful acupuncturists had inscribed bones and tortoise shells with symbols representing their medical knowledge. At roughly the same time, methods for casting bronze were developed, and needles made of this alloy began to appear. Still later, between what is known as the Warring States Period (465–221 B.C.) and the Western Han Dynasty (206 B.C.–A.D. 24), iron needles were created. These successfully displaced stone as the instrument of choice.

One hundred years later, around A.D. 100, needles of gold and silver were constructed. At least nine different shapes of needles were made, each for different purposes. Some needles, those that were sharp and thin, were used specifically for puncturing. Others, blunt and thick instruments, were used for massage. By this time, the ideas of yin and yang, the Five Element Theory, moxibustion, and the concepts of pulse, blood, chi, shen, and channels were firmly incorporated into the medical knowledge of the time.

or to relieve certain abdominal pains. Since there are not any accessible points near the large intestine itself, the practitioner will have to select an

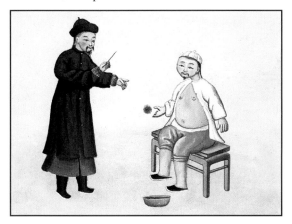

available point, such as the Hegu point (Large Intestine number four; also Ho-Ku, He Gu) found on the web of skin between the thumb and forefinger. This point can be manipulated either with a needle, with heat, or simply with pressure to relieve the blockage and restore the flow of chi to a healthy level.

針灸

Acupuncture and the Modern World

For many years, acupuncture was not well received by the established medical community in the developed world. It was frowned upon and considered to be the product of superstition and tradition. Traditional Chinese medicine practitioners have felt that Western medical doctors dismissed their methods without fair consideration, while Western medical associations have complained about the lack of empirical evidence to support acupuncturists' claims of successful healing.

Today, however, acupuncture is used throughout the world by health care professionals of all types. In some countries, such as France, acupuncturists must become licensed medical doctors before practicing acupuncture. In the United States, not all states have licensing procedures for acupuncturists, and requirements vary greatly among the states that do have them.

Research Shows Acupuncture's Effectiveness

Numerous research groups worldwide have been investigating acupuncture from a scientific perspective. Research indicates that there is indeed some validity to the practice. The World Health Organization (WHO) reports that significant advances have been made in the scientific understanding of the processes involved in acupuncture. Clinical studies have demonstrated that acupuncture analgesia can be used effectively during surgery and in the treatment of severe and chronic pain. Other studies have indicated that the acupuncture process may indeed regulate body functions and enhance the immune system.

UCLA's Center for East-West Medicine also notes that "Research implicating a role for neurotransmitters such as serotonin, norepinephrine, dopamine, prostaglandins and the endogenous opioids may help explain acupuncture's ability to effect change in pain and other physiological pathways. While it is true that this technique is best known to be effective in the treatment of many painful conditions, it is also used widely in the management of many other conditions in China and in many parts of the world. These include asthma, stress, depression, anxiety, women's health problems, gastrointestinal discomfort and neurological disorders including post-stroke rehabilitation. Acupuncture has been used in the operating room in conjunction with chemical agents to allow for safer and less painful surgical procedures. There is also some research and clinical evidence of its effectiveness against drug, alcohol and nicotine addiction."

Bruce Pomeranz, a Canadian neurophysiologist, has been studying acupuncture for twenty years. His research has led him to believe that acupuncture reduces pain by triggering the release of endorphins, the body's natural painkillers; ACTH (adrenocorticotropic hormone), a hormone that helps fight inflammation; and prostaglandins, which help wounds to heal. Other research teams have supported the endorphin theory. And some researchers theorize that acupuncture points may have electrical properties that, when stimulated, alter chemical neurotransmitters in the body as well as altering the body's natural electrical currents or electromagnetic fields. According to the World Health Organization, laboratory results and clinical trials have shown that acupuncture treatment could remarkably regulate the number of natural killer cells, T-lymphocytes, B-cells, and the level of IgG and IgA.

Because there has been sufficient current research suggesting the positive benefits of acupuncture, many medical organizations and insurance companies have been prompted to reevaluate their positions on the practice.

針灸

Additional Techniques Used in Traditional Chinese Medicine

Acupressure

Sometimes acupoints are stimulated using techniques other than acupuncture needles.

Hands, for instance, have been used as healing tools since the beginning of time. Acupressure uses the fingers or palms rather than needles to apply pressure to acupoints. Entire channels can also be massaged in the hope of freeing the blocked energy within, promoting the flow of chi, and restoring good health. There are many systems of therapeutic massage, including Shiatsu, Jin Shin Do, and Tibetan massage.

Different oils are often used with massage techniques, and their proper use is associated with the seasons. Olive and sesame oils are used in winter while sandalwood oil can be used in summer. Some customs avoid massage altogether during the summer months.

Moxibustion

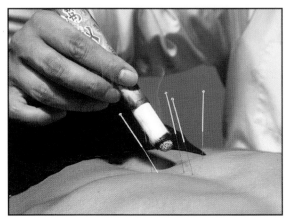

Moxibustion is a healing practice that uses mugwort *(Artemisia vulgaris)*, an herb, to form cones called moxa. These cones are ignited and placed either directly on the surface of the skin over a suitable acupuncture point or on some insulating material first. Moxa is thought to be pure yang energy, and it is capable not only of restoring prenatal chi but also of opening all the acupuncture channels and suppressing a great number of diseases.

The Healing Art of Chi Kung

Chi kung techniques are held in high esteem in China. In fact, when its political leaders hold their annual conference, exceptional chi kung masters are invited to treat them. These treatments are usually done in two parts. In the first, the practitioner projects chi into the body of the client without any physical contact. Using a special form of chi, known as spiral or penetrating chi, advanced practitioners can project this substance as far as 16 feet.

Chi kung is considered essential to conditioning the body to resist disease. It is believed to promote health, well-being, and longevity and is used to treat a variety of chronic diseases and conditions, including anxiety, hypertension, depression, and heart disease. Chi kung is practiced by great numbers of people in China, and every day it is common to see a chi kung master instructing hundreds of people out of doors. In this way, people who practice assume the responsibility for their own health and well-being before they become ill.

針灸

Balancing Energy—the Traditional Goal

Restoring the body to its natural balance is the goal of every traditional physician. Every therapeutic tool, every diagnostic strategy is designed to reveal the movements of energy and the processes of change or stagnation within the body. The physician works to restore us to health, to a state of wholeness, balance, and well-being. But, as we have seen, it is possible for us to accomplish this for ourselves. Tai chi chuan is an art devoted to just this goal.

To a Westerner, traditional Chinese medicine seems almost quaint compared to the ultrasophisticated scientific medicine to which we are accustomed. This is largely because the methods still rely on ancient philosophical terms and concepts for expression. This handicap, however, does not negate a central underlying fact concerning this Chinese medical system: Its methods are not only highly effective in many cases, but they are also relatively inexpensive and available to virtually everyone who is in need. Traditional Chinese medical practitioners have an uncanny ability to point out habits and conditions in our lives that cause weakness and disease. They are able not only to diagnose a problem, but suggest causes, prescribe time-honored treatments, recommend specific dietary changes including what and when to eat and drink, and even suggest lifestyle changes.

The doctor works systematically, using simple but effective methods that have withstood the test of time. In a culture with limited financial and scientific resources, a medical system that relies on inexpensive, readily available tools and therapeutic prescriptions that anyone can follow is absolutely priceless. This is one major reason why traditional medical techniques continue to thrive throughout much of the world.

Tai Chi
Chuan

太極

One day the Taoist monk Chang San-feng was disturbed by the sounds of a snake and a crane fighting in his court-yard. Each time the crane's rapierlike beak stabbed, the flexible snake twisted out of reach. And the crane's wings, like shields, protected its long neck from the snake's striking head. According to the myth, from observing this battle, Chang San-feng developed the art of tai chi chuan, which is based on the concept of yielding in the face of aggression.

WISDOM OF TAI CHI

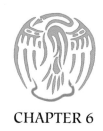

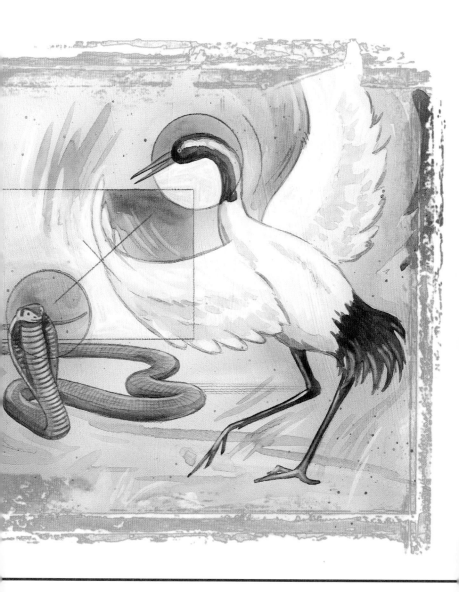

CHAPTER 6

太極
The Myth

As we have seen, the images conveyed in the telling of a myth lend themselves well to the spirit and the ideas of tai chi chuan. For this reason, many myths have sprung up around the art of tai chi and its principal actors, and Chang San-feng figures prominently in many of them. Another famous myth depicts Chang San-feng seeking the fabled elixir of life, a liquid formula that reputedly makes one immortal. One night, while in a deep sleep after an exhausting search for the elixir, the movements of tai chi chaun were revealed to him in a dream.

After careful reflection, it occurred to him that perhaps the secret of the elixir was related to these movements. It dawned on him that the idea of drinking the elixir of immortality was actually an allegory in which the set of tai chi exercises revealed in the dream represented the formula for the elixir itself. He noted that chi in the body exhibited a number of properties similar to liquids. It flows, for example, through the many acupuncture channels. He also noted that when the chi flows in abundance, good health prevails, and when it is blocked, illness soon follows.

Like water, chi in the body can also be affected by certain natural forces, such as the gravitational pull of the moon. He finally realized that the liquid elixir could actually represent chi. By performing the movements revealed to him, Chang San-feng concluded, he would be developing chi and incorporating it into his body as an essential life- and health-giving force.

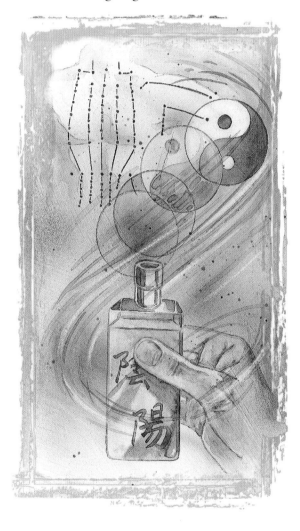

太極

Taoism—the Roots of Tai Chi Chuan

While we will never know whether Chang San-feng's initial inspiration actually came from the fight between the snake and the crane or from a dream, we do know that this twelfth century Taoist based his invention of tai chi chuan movements on the fundamental principles of Lao Tzu and Taoism. As noted in Chapter 1, tai chi chuan means "perfect boxing," and it refers to a martial art based upon the philosophical principles of Taoism. As suggested in Chang San-feng's dream, this art also bestows upon its practitioners the remarkable benefits of health and well-being. When mastered, the art, through its graceful yet practical movements, is a living expression of harmony as applied to life and to each encounter with the ten thousand things of the Tao. Every action is used to bring about perfect balance with the forces encountered in the world, and so, the art can be said actually to teach its practitioners how to apply the principle of yin and yang.

Just as tai chi chuan is a practice devoted to dealing with the forces of the physical world, it also seeks to develop the mind. It does so not by treating mind and body as separate parts, but as a single cohesive unit. The exercises, then, were designed not only for the body, but also for the mind. Strengthening one means strengthening the other. At its highest levels, tai chi chuan is also part of a Taoist spiritual discipline that seeks to elevate the mind and purify the body.

太極

The Living Iconography of Tai Chi

Tai chi movements represent specific philosophical principles. Some even believe that the art of tai chi was intended as a means of passing down highly specialized knowledge—that is, the basic principles of Taoism. Realizing the passion of many young men for testing their strength through fighting and their typical aversion to scholasticism, past masters conceived of a brilliant plan. To save their wisdom from completely disappearing with the passage of centuries, they embedded it in the movements of tai chi. Further, the belief is that they made the art irresistibly appealing by endowing it with all of the qualities necessary to be a great fighter. Learning to fight, then, necessitated learning all of the Taoist principles—a clever scheme indeed, and one that has worked very well.

Whether or not there is any truth to this belief, each move is, in fact, an icon that represents specific ideas. Together the postures form something of an esoteric dance that weaves knowledge and movements together so cleverly that only someone deeply versed in Taoist philosophy can interpret them accurately. Knowledgeable viewers who understand the moves, however, can provide extensive commentaries on both internal healing effects and combat applications. Such commentators can also discuss the philosophical underpinnings of the movements.

The names of different moves in tai chi, like the names of the cards in a Tarot deck, are a way of organizing information and describe categories with their own unique purpose. (See "The Iconography of Tarot," page 202.) For this reason, the tai chi moves can be considered icons. When linked together in a complete set of tai chi movements, the icons act as a living library for students to imitate, study, and contemplate.

太極

The History: Wu T'ang Mountain

The actual history and development of tai chi chuan is at least as mysterious as that of Taoism, the philosophy that gave it birth. Whether the original set of movements, called forms, were divinely inspired or whether they were developed through the painstaking research of generations of martial artists has never really been answered. It is very likely that no one will ever know the whole story.

Some say Chang San-feng was a hermit and an alchemist. Others believe he was a monk. Most likely, he was a monk knowledgeable in the secret practices of Taoism such as chi kung. Whatever he was, there is little doubt that sometime around A.D. 1200, together with a small group of disciples, he founded two Taoist temples. One, called the White Clouded Temple, was built on Beijing West Mountain to teach meditation and Taoism. The other, called Wu T'ang Temple, was built on Wu T'ang Mountain in Hupei Province specifically to teach tai chi and related disciplines.

Whether or not Chang San-feng actually created the art of tai chi, however, has been the subject of great debate. *The Ningpo Chronicle*, a record of the time, lists the names of some martial arts postures still in use in tai chi practice today. This suggests that the art was in existence then. Other records indicate that the art was passed on to Yeh Chi-mei, a native of Ningpo. Taken together, the two old records appear to confirm that Chang San-feng at least knew the art at the time.

Prior to Chang San-feng's discovery, the main system of martial arts was *(continued on page 204)*

THE ICONOGRAPHY OF
TAROT

Some believe that the deck of cards known as the Tarot, and even its contemporary derivative, our 52-card playing deck, are actually repositories of highly specialized information. Ancient Egyptian priests reasoned correctly that their wisdom would survive the ages only if it was preserved in a form that appealed to most people.

The Tarot deck, then, was created to serve two purposes. Recognizing greed as a perennial human weakness, they designed the cards so they could be used as a gambling tool. In this capacity they have been used with unquestionable success ever since. On a more significant level, however, the cards describe archetypal figures or situations well-known in Western thought. Some of these are The Magician, Nature, Temptation, The Sphinx, The Sun, and The World.

Today many different Tarot decks have been created to serve various purposes. Each of these describes significant events and symbols in a particular system of knowledge or culture. Tarot decks are now associated with Tibetan Buddhism, the Maya, and other civilizations such as that of the Native Americans. An analysis of the symbolism behind the cards of any one system does, in fact, reveal a very elaborate system of knowledge.

The Right-Turning Conch Shell, a card from the Tibetan deck, is one of Eight Symbols of Good Fortune and is associated with the hope that the Buddhist scriptures, the wisdom teachings, will be dis-

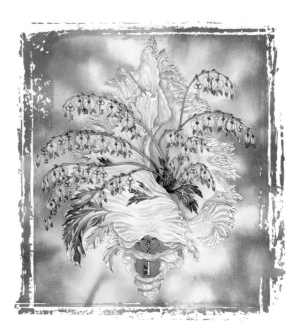

seminated everywhere, in all directions, like the sound made by a conch shell trumpet.

The right-turning conch shell is among the oldest of all ritual objects. Its use predates fabricated ritual objects since it could, from time to time, be found in nature. Most conch shells have a spiral shape that turns to the left. Those that turn right are rare, and consequently, even today they are highly prized.

These shells are sometimes used as ritual ornaments, as instruments for making musical offerings (the trumpet sound), to summon the congregation, and to decorate a throne or an alter. In divination, this card suggests increasing fame and wealth. When handled by a Tibetan monk, the shell evokes these and other meanings that of the Shaolin school, introduced by Bodhidharma more than 600 years earlier. Since Shaolin techniques relied heavily on physical strength and bravery, it was known as a "hard" school of self-defense and was considered to be an external system, one that relied on skill coupled with physical prowess. The art of tai chi, however, suggested a completely different fight-

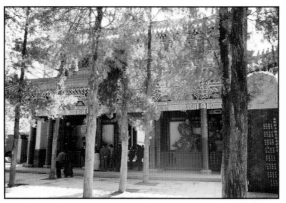

The Shaolin Temple

ing strategy, one that required the development of a special form of awareness that links body and mind and uses a passive energy developed through the application of special techniques. For these reasons, tai chi came to be thought of as an internal or mental system that relied on "soft" self-defense techniques. Many tai chi historians believe that these soft techniques were completely unknown at the time.

True to Lao Tzu's *Tao Te Ching*, the monk's methods relied on the yin forces of passivity and the ability to yield when confronted by the aggressive forces of the yang. By bending, says the *Tao Te Ching*, we can avoid breaking. If we are bent, we can straighten. Once broken, though, we remain broken.

Yang Lu-ch'uan and the Theft of Tai Chi

Tai chi's history is a tale of subterfuge and deceit, but also of wisdom and forgiveness. Until modern times, it was virtually impossible to learn the discipline unless one had a close association with the family of a master who taught it. Those who knew the secrets of tai chi guarded them carefully, as this knowledge was a great source of power and authority. As a result, there was considerable rivalry between many of these tai chi masters. Independent masters passed on the knowledge of tai chi only to their sons and other highly privileged family members or associates. And masters affiliated with Taoist temples only taught tai chi to other temple members. Temple secrets, like family secrets, were carefully guarded. It is said, for example, that there were only two ways out of a Shaolin temple: Either the monks carried you out feet first or they let you out, something that did not often happen.

Sometime early in the nineteenth century a well-known boxer, Yang Lu-ch'uan, decided he needed to learn tai chi to improve his art. His previous martial training had been conducted in the

YANG THE UNBEATABLE DEFEATS THE SHAOLIN PRIESTS

Favorite tai chi stories often recount the defeat of an arrogant or troublesome martial artist at the hands of a great tai chi master. Typically the master uses an absolute minimum of force to defeat powerful opponents by propelling them many feet away. The following story describes such a defeat of the Taoists' archrivals, the Shaolin priests.

One warm summer afternoon, after a long walk, Yang Lu-ch'an was resting quietly on the banks of a slowly moving river. Just behind him, two Shaolin priests were following the road to town. Knowing his reputation, these priests would normally have shown him every courtesy. But seeing the great fighter resting by the stream and supposing him to be half asleep, they decided to play a trick on him. Creeping up from behind, they wanted to throw him into the river, just to get him wet and ruin his reputation.

Yang the Unbeatable, however, was not sleeping at all; he was in a state of complete attention, practicing his Taoist breathing techniques. All his senses were completely awakened, and he actually heard the two men approaching. Just as they pounced, Yang Lu-ch'an stood up and moved into a tai chi posture. With an almost imperceptible movement of his back and shoulders, he threw the two attackers far into the river. The priests swam to the other side, continuing their journey from a safer, more respectful distance.

"hard," external techniques of the Buddhists' Shaolin temple. Being a fighter, Yang Lu-ch'an must have battled taichiists, as practitioners of tai chi are sometimes called, since he recognized the value of their "soft," internal Taoist method. In it he saw a complement to his own style.

The most famous independent tai chi instructor at the time was Chen Chang Shen, and Yang Lu-ch'an hoped to study with him. Realizing that he could not approach the master as a boxer seeking special instruction, he took a position in the household as a servant. Each evening, the story goes, he crept up to the keyhole and secretly watched the master instructing his family members. Later at night, when the house was quiet, Yang Lu-ch'an would practice. Unfortunately, because he was not under the direct instruction of Chen Chang Shen, he learned only the movements themselves, not their martial applications. Learning these required verbal tutelage directly from the master.

The old master, however, was well aware of the spy. Had he revealed what he knew to the rest of his family, there is little doubt that the intruder would have been put to death or at least have lost a hand. One night, Chen Chang Shen turned the tables and spied on Yang Lu-ch'an when he was practicing. Recognizing the great potential in this servant-impostor, the master proceeded, over the next few years, to teach him everything he knew. Under the master's patronage and protection, Yang Lu-ch'an then challenged each of the fighters in the family, defeating them each in their turn. After leaving the Chen household for Beijing, he successfully defeated the 18 most prominent martial artists in the country. As a result, he was given the title, "Yang the Unbeatable." "Old Master Yang," as he was later called, became something of a legend in his own time, and there are many wonderful stories about his exploits.

Yang taught tai chi to his own three sons and other trusted associates. He was also invited to teach the art to the Royal Court and to certain branches of the military. This new Yang style of tai chi was also taught to the Wu family, where it gradually became yet another distinct style. Interestingly, one of Yang Lu-ch'an's descendants, his grandson Yang Ch'eng Fu (1883–1935), popularized tai chi and, in a radical departure from tradition, made the art available to the general public. Today there are many tai chi styles, but the styles of the three families—Chen, Yang, and Wu—are among the most common.

太極

The Written Record

Books about tai chi and tai chi practice did not become available to the general public until the beginning of the twentieth century. Until that time, students always received personal instruction in a master's home or temple. There was no need for written materials because the instructions were delivered orally. The laborious process of wood block printing also discouraged creating written documents about tai chi, and so very few were written.

There are, however, eight texts dating from the early tai chi masters that are known as "The Classics." Of these, three are collectively referred to as *The Tai Chi Bible*. In their entirety, all eight volumes comprise only a few thousand words. Nevertheless, it is on the basis of these master works, and the subsequent commentaries, that tai chi is practiced today.

The first book, *The Book of Tai Chi Chuan,* is attributed by convention to Chang San-feng himself. It emphasizes the form and discusses in some detail how a practitioner should move when practicing. The second text, *Treatise of Tai Chi Chuan,* is attributed to another legendary character, Wang Chen-yeuh. This work focuses on the underlying philosophical principles of tai chi. It also discusses the martial applications of the art. The third text is the *Elucidation of the Thirteen Postures.* Some believe this text also was written by Wang Chen-yeuh, but others think it was written by an academically inclined tai chi master named Wu Yu-hsiang. This book centers on the inner processes of tai chi and focuses on the idea of chi and its functions as they apply to the art. The other texts include *Song of the Thir-*

teen *Postures*, by Wu Yu-hsiang, *Song of Push Hands*, by an unknown author, *Five Character Secret*, by Li I-yu, *Essentials of the Practice of the Form* and *Push Hands*, by Li I-yu, and *Yang's Ten Important Points*, by Yang Cheng-fu.

The Five Character Secret

The classic *The Five Character Secret*, written by Li I-yu, describes the nature of tai chi and, in a sense, lays bare its heart and soul. The Chinese language differs from English in this important respect: Each word is represented by a distinct character. Rather than using separate letters to form a particular word, it has its own unique symbol. So the five characters in the title of the classic refer to five words: calm, agility, breath, internal force, and spirit. These five terms are intended to represent the essence of tai chi practice. An interpretation of the salient ideas of *The Five Character Secret* is presented below.

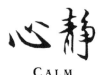

CALM

The Chinese have a special word, *hsin*, meaning heart-mind. It refers to a mental intention that has not yet been expressed. The disposition of hsin must be calm; otherwise it will not be possible to concentrate. Without concentration, our movements and actions will lack direction and be uncertain. If we are calm, we can use the mind to match our opponent's moves perfectly. What is important is that we realize our situation and are ready to deal with opposition as it unfolds. We can only realize this by evaluating our own circumstances, then considering them objectively and dispassionately. If we become emotionally involved or begin to react based on our expectations rather than to the events themselves, we will not be masters of the situation.

AGILITY

Agility refers to coordinating all body parts at once. When we advance or retreat, the body must respond immediately to the requirements of the moment. This is only possible if there is a continuous link between every part of the body, particularly the legs and waist. If the linkage is not present, the chi cannot flow smoothly, and as a result, we will be clumsy. The secret to agility is this: At first do not follow the ideas issued by your own mind. Instead, follow the exact movements of your opponent. Later, after your body knows how to follow, you will be able to follow both your mind and the movements of the opponent. But skill such as this takes time to develop.

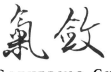

GATHERING CHI

If we learn how to concentrate the chi by using our mind, we will have an advantage over our opponent. When the chi is concentrated, for example, even our breathing patterns become powerful tools. Breathing in, in concert with the intention of the mind, has the power to upset the balance of the opponent. Breathing out, in concert with the mind, has the power to weaken the opponent. Remember, these forces work through the action of the chi and not through muscular strength.

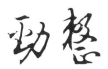

INTERNAL FORCE

With practice, it is possible to produce an internal energy known as *chin* (see pages 216–220). To use this force, however, it is first necessary to create it and then to move it up from the feet, to amplify it in the legs, to direct it at the waist, and then move it to the arms and discharge it through the fingers. To accomplish this feat, the timing must be impeccable, so that there is not a single uncoordinated move. Over time, the chin, when applied, becomes as smooth flowing and irresistible as the flow of a tide.

SPIRIT: THE SPIRIT OF VITALITY

The spirit of vitality, an aspect of spirit, is the last of the five secrets. It can only be possessed if the other four are already mastered. Possessing this ability enables the practitioner to demonstrate applications of the two polarities, the yin and the yang, and to practice at the very high level of collecting and emitting chi. When we collect chi, it moves downward from the shoulders and collects in the abdominal region. When we emit chi, it moves up from the abdomen, through the spine, to the shoulders, into the arms, and out the fingers. If we are able to collect chi, then we are said to understand yin energy. If we can emit chi, then we are said to understand yang energy.

If these five ideas are understood properly and put into daily practice, they will help ensure success in learning the art of tai chi chuan. If they are ignored, the masters tell us there is very little hope in ever achieving a high level of proficiency. Further, the mastery of each principle can be regarded as a goal that, when achieved, becomes a landmark.

太極

The Postures

Each of the movements in tai chi is known as a posture or a move. When these moves are connected, they are called a form or a set. Over time, under the guidance of master practitioners, many different forms have developed. All of them, however, rely on the same underlying principles.

It is likely that tai chi is the series of rhythmic dancelike movements we know today because of its relationship to the martial arts. Some believe that the exercises originally were simply a series of unconnected postures used exclusively to maintain health. This may well be the case, since many systems of exercises, such as some types of chi kung and yoga, rely almost entirely on standing, seated, or prone postures. While these systems can be very rhythmic in themselves, there is no question that tai chi can clearly be distinguished from the others by its involvement with the movement of the feet and legs.

At the same time, tai chi does not sacrifice the meditative spirit common to some forms of yoga. In fact, the art of tai chi chuan is considered a moving meditation. The central difference between a seated meditation and tai chi is that in tai chi, the entire body, including all the internal organs, muscles, tendons, and limbs, work together.

The movements themselves and the way they are linked together are very strictly organized, and dedicated practice under expert tutelage is required to master the finer points governing them. Since the tradition is so old, it has been refined by generations of instructors. Through

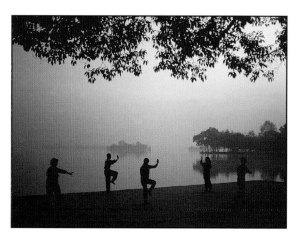

trial and error during hand-to-hand combat and through careful analysis, tai chi has been developed to the point where, regardless of the particular training school, there is a set of universal principles held to be true by the majority of schools.

Typically, these principles are learned as the movements themselves are taught. Instruction is simultaneously mental and physical, a convenient structure for students because learning becomes a step-by-step process in which intellectual knowledge always corresponds to a physical exercise. This means that intellectual development will not exceed physical development. Long forms of tai chi naturally take a longer period to learn since they are composed of many more movements. A long form may contain 60, 108, or even 150 movements, while a shorter form might have only 27 movements. Aside from the health benefits and martial applications, one of the great joys of learning this art is that there seems to be no end to its depth. This means that taichiists are continuously challenged to improve their art.

太極
Chin and the Concept of Intrinsic Energy

Earlier we described chi as the life force found throughout creation. The ability to collect chi from the universe and to move chi throughout the body to every tissue is something chi kung practitioners and taichiists learn to do. It happens naturally, simply by practicing. We have also discussed the idea of cultivating shen, meaning spirit, which requires a mastery of both the emotions and the intellect. There is a third force, known as chin. Together with the chi and shen, chin forms a trinity known as the internal energies. From these basic energies, a number of other forces are generated by the tai chi practitioner. In fact, by some accounts, more than 35 distinct energies can be cultivated and used in tai chi applications. These energies are unique to tai chi, and they are applied in association with the eight elements and the five phases.

Chin (also called jin or jing) is another force like chi and shen that can only be used effectively through practice. When practitioners use chin, they are using a substance created by the action of shen in relation to the chi. Once taichiists can move chin through their bodies, they can begin to apply it in different martial situations such as in the movements related to the five phases.

To understand how chin might be applied, we must first identify its characteristics. Chin is an internal force unlike the external force called *li* generated by the muscles. Tai chi theory maintains that li is related to and generated from the bones and muscles. In particular, it is related to the area of the upper body around the shoulder blades. Li is the raw yang energy taichiists try to avoid using since it is antithetical to chin energy.

Chin, on the other hand, is a special energy that is formed when the tendons and sinews around the bones are actually relaxed. This is one reason why tai chi theory stresses the importance of relaxing the many different muscle groups in the body and eliminating any unnecessary tension. Chin energy has often been likened to the energy that issues from the tip of a bull whip. Following a spiral movement of delivery, the energy is concentrated along an ever-narrowing ribbon of leather until it is expressed with great force and flawless precision at the delicate tip.

Another principle difference is that li is the strength derived from the upper body, whereas chin is the force native to the lower body. Exactly how we are to summon chin and how we can direct its flow is described in this paraphrased fourth verse of Chang San-feng's *Tai Chi Chuan Ching*.

> The root of the chin should be in
>   the feet.
> It flows upward following the legs.
> Directed by the waist,
> Chin is presented through the fingers.

Understanding this short verse, however, is not as straightforward as it might seem, and it has prompted endless commentaries. Interpreting it properly presupposes a certain knowledge of tai chi basics. Root, for example, is an idea related to a special sense of balance. When a practitioner is said to be rooted, the image conveyed is one of the deep roots of a huge tree extending far below the surface of the earth. These effectively ground the taichiist, making a stable platform for the forthcoming action.

The root is related to the yongquan acupoint, which is located on one of the 12 main acupuncture channels, the Kidney Channel. The point

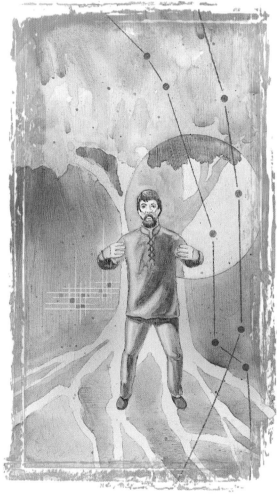

name means gushing spring, and the imagery associated with it describes the flow of chi. The chi is abundant at this acupoint, as indicated by the gushing water analogy. Massaging this point will encourage the flow of chi either into or out of the body, and people who visit chi kung masters often experience the chi as a breeze moving out of their bodies at the yongquan point.

As we have seen, though, chi is not chin. Chin does not exist unless it is created by the taichiist, and it is dependent upon the forces of both chi and shen as well. So the taichiist must first create chin by using the spirit—shen—and the life force—chi.

The verse does not specifically mention that it is only at the command of the mind, known as the "I" in Chinese, that the chin can begin to circulate. But, in fact, it is at the taichiist's mental direction that the chin is first created and then moved from its root in the feet, up through the body.

As it moves upward, the chin gains momentum, like the energy moving along the ever narrowing bull whip. When it reaches the hips, the waist begins to move at the exact moment when it can gain the most leverage. Like a pivot, it swings into the position decided upon beforehand by the taichiist. Continuing upward, the chin gathers yet more momentum as it moves up the spine, through the back and shoulders, along the arms, past the elbows and finally out the fingers. The entire movement is coordinated, so that each part of the body acts together with the others.

太極

Martial Application of Tai Chi:

The Eight Postures & the Five Phases

We have seen how the Wu Chi gives birth to the yin and the yang and how the interaction of these primal energies creates the eight forces of nature: heaven, earth, lake, mountain, wind, thunder, water, and fire. In the chapter on traditional Chinese medicine, we also discussed a second theory, known as the Five Element Theory. This theory is also called the Five Phase Theory because the relationship between the elements is expressed as the movement or transformation demonstrated in the diagram of the cycles of destruction and creation. *(See pages 226–227.)*

When the symbols for the eight forces of nature are coupled with those of the five phases, thirteen configurations result. These formations are related to thirteen fundamental tai chi ideas. These include eight distinct martial techniques that are applied within five sets of movements.

The Eight Techniques and Their Trigrams

We saw in Chapter 1 how the original eight trigrams are used to form the hexagrams of the *I Ching* and how they correspond to the three levels of existence: The uppermost line represents heaven; the middle line, humanity; and the lowest line, earth. These trigrams are very ancient and even predate the creation of the *I Ching*. The idea behind the trigrams is attributed to the mythical ruler Fu Hsi who lived more than 5,000 years ago during the early era when hunting and fishing were the primary occupations. When the elements are organized into opposing pairs and associated with the points of the compass, the arrangement is known as the "Sequence of Earlier Heaven" or sometimes as "The Primal Arrangement." Heaven and earth are associated with south and north, mountain and lake with northwest and southeast, fire and water with the east and west, and, thunder and wind with the northeast and southwest.

From this basic structure, tai chi chuan uses the trigrams as a means of representing information. Eight fighting techniques, movements known as the "Eight Gates," are assigned to particular trigrams. Like the elements themselves, the movements are organized into complementary and opposing pairs of yang and yin grouped as follows; ward off and roll back, press and push, pull down and split, elbow stroke and shoulder stroke.

Since these movements are associated with an element, they are also associated with a direction and are arranged in pairs of complementary opposites around the Tai Chi symbol. The eight trigrams are divided into two halves, known as the four cardinal directions (S, N, E, W) and the four corners (SE, NE, SW, NW).

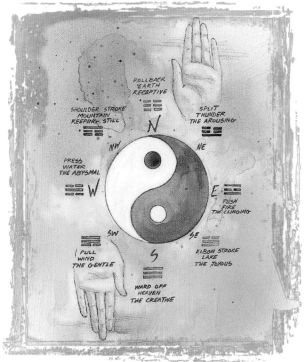

The Eight Elements

The south is the location of heaven. It is represented by three yang lines, indicating the greatest concentration of yang chi in the entire system.

In terms of tai chi, this translates into the most powerful and aggressive force. When coupled with the creativity associated with heaven, it becomes the epitome of intelligently applied force. The tai chi movement associated with this hexagram is known as ward off.

The north is the direction of earth. This is the trigram of roll back, the complement to ward off. True to theory, rollback is denoted by three broken lines. Rather than seeking to confront, this move indicates a retreat. By yielding strategically, the target disappears and the efforts of the opponent are diffused harmlessly. In ward off and roll back we again see the pattern of advance and yield, of the hard and the soft; two forces that are fully equal, each unmatchable in its own right.

Press, indicated by the trigram for water, is assigned to the west. It is signified by two broken lines with a solid line between. Its complement, push, symbolized by fire, is found in the east. This trigram is two solid lines separated by a broken line.

The four corners are represented in the northeast by thunder and its movement, split, and in the southwest by wind and its movement, pull. Mountain is located in the northwest. Its movement is the shoulder stroke. Lake, its complement, is in the southeast. Its move is an elbow stroke. When arranged with their attributes on the points of a compass, the techniques appear as in the diagram on page 223.

As you might imagine, applying these techniques is not a simple matter. First of all, each of the moves indicated by the eight trigrams must be learned. A push, for example, does not mean simply pushing someone away or down with brute force. The action refers to a detailed sequence of movements executed in a precise way. Further, each of the eight moves can be found in several different places in the complete set of tai chi postures.

The Five Phases

As we have seen in the chapter on traditional Chinese medicine, the Five Element Theory is yet another important Taoist theory. It has also been incorporated into tai chi chuan. To avoid confusing it with the eight elements, we will refer to it here by its other name, the Five Phase Theory. Because of their inherent qualities, five elements—earth, fire, water, metal, and wood—were selected by the ancient sages to describe patterns and relationships between many variables. We also saw, in the last chapter, how they relate to one another in an abstract sense and how they can be used to describe the relationship between the seasons. In tai chi chuan, they are used to describe five special movements, five different weapons, and five different energies. They are also a tool for tactical planning.

Tai chi theory maintains that knowledge of the five phases will lead to an advantage since its principles can be used in either tactical advance or tactical retreat. The phases also give us insight into the intention of the opponent. This intellectual advantage is the reason tai chi is considered an internal art: Superior reasoning, it is believed, has the advantage over superior strength. Using the phases, we can actually "see" the other's plan before it is executed. In its essence, the information reveals an opponent's moves beforehand so they can be countered.

Such skill is often bewildering to the casual observer. Since knowledge of the phases enables us to "predict" the tactics of others, in the past the art was often considered to be some kind of Taoist "magic." Really, however, these techniques rely on a knowledge of anatomy, on the mechanics of movements, and sophisticated insights into methods of tactical planning. There is an interesting parallel here between the martial foresight of a taichiist and the psychological intuitions achieved by study of the *I Ching*.

The relationships among the five phases are represented by a circle that has five points. One line is drawn around the circumference of these points. This represents one set of relationships known as the constructive cycle used in defense. In this sequence, we find water supporting wood, wood supporting fire, fire supporting earth, and earth supporting water. This suggests the sequence of moves that might be used in a tactical retreat. Another line is drawn within the circle in the shape of a pentagram, which represents a second set of relationships known as the destructive cycle used in offensive tactics. In this sequence, we find water destroying fire, which vanquishes metal, which, in its turn, subdues wood, and so on. The

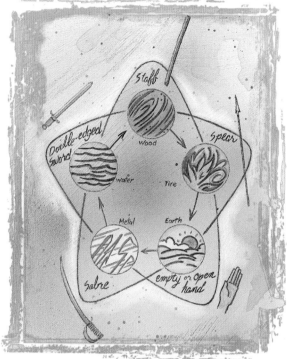

The Five Phase Theory

diagram above outlines these two patterns of relationships. They are important because they suggest particular movements and form the basis of tai chi strategy in combat.

There is a third set of relationships, however, and so another unique diagram must be created. In this second diagram, four points are located on the perimeter, and one is placed in the middle. This diagram is related to the five tactical movements used in tai chi. Known as advance, retreat, step and gaze left, step and look right, and central balance, these movements are related to the Five Phase Theory.

Not all tai chi masters, though, agree about which elements are related to which movements. One very common set of correspondences has fire relating to advance, water to retreat, metal to step and look left, wood to step and look right, and earth to central balance.

In this scheme, earth is accorded a very prominent position. It is recognized as the mother of all others, and so it is given the center position. In the same way that earth is considered the locus of the other elements, central balance to which earth corresponds is thought to be the fulcrum on which all other movements depend. For a practitioner, this suggests that cultivating central balance is a prerequisite to mastering the other movements.

太極

Tai Chi Weaponry

The ideas behind the phases and their relationships also apply to five weapons. Just as the elements represent the inner quality of each movement, they play the *(continued on page 232)*

CHINESE SYMBOLISM OF
THE SWORD

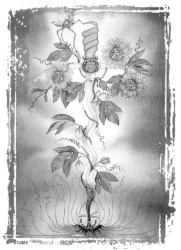

Magicians in ancient China were reputed to have driven off demons with swords. There also were swords forged out of the kidney and liver of a mythological hare from the Kuenlun Mountains. And in keeping with the Taoist philosophy of the opposing forces of yin and yang, swords were said to have been either feminine or masculine. Of the five tai chi weapons realted to the five phases, the two-edged sword represents water, a feminine element.

The symbolism in the painting of the passion flower reflects much of our study of tai chi. The sword emerges from the heart of a flower and supports the plant as it climbs. At its full height, a circle contains the five points that relate to the five phases. The mantis, which is well known to martial artists as an insect with special fighting abilities, awaits its prey in a state of compete calm.

MASTER CHANG SAN-FENG AND THE TRANSMISSION OF THE T'AI CHI SPEAR

Master Chang San-feng, considered to be an Immortal, loved to go to the Wu T'ang Mountains near his temple and ponder life. He meandered among great trees, always cultivating his relationship with the forest and its inhabitants. His favorite time was morning, when he would climb the highest peak and sit in meditation with the rising sun. At this time of day, as the light shifted from a soft glow to brilliant sky, he would practice chi kung.

At an early hour one day, as the fog still clung to the mountains, Master Chang was enraptured by a brilliant light in the distant sky. Spellbound, he watched as the light spiraled and pulsed, then descended. Waking from his trance, he rushed into the woods thinking he could find the very place where the light seemed to touch the land. Upon reaching what seemed to be just the place, he came upon a mountain cave. At the cave entrance were two snakes with eyes of fire. The Immortal summoned light from the Heavens, and the snakes transformed into two long spears. Their properties were mysterious. Although they seemed to be wooden, they were not made from any known tree. These spears could be rigid or flexible, soft or hard, and long or short at his command.

The Immortal then noticed another light glowing from the cave. Beyond the spears he saw a book, entitled T'ai Chi Stick-Adhere Spear, which he retrieved with great interest. Within its pages were poems and

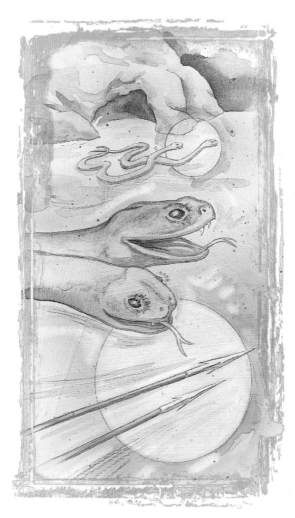

songs telling the mysteries of the spear that no mortal could understand. But Master Chang, Immortal that he was, could understand everything in the little text. He transformed the great secrets of the spear into a set of postures so that he could share this treasure with the world. And that is how we came to have the knowledge of the spear today.

same role for weapons. It can be said that there is a partnership between each movement and its allied weapon. Each pair has distinct applications, and these are related to particular tactics in hand-to-hand combat.

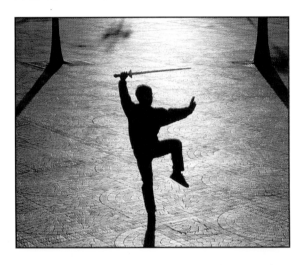

In terms of the weapons themselves, earth is represented by an empty hand, metal by a saber, wood by a staff, water by a two-edged sword, and fire by a spear. In the same way that earth is thought of as mother to the other elements, all weapons are considered to be descendants of the empty hand. In action, the natural ability of the open hand is grasping. It can control the two-edged sword if it can grasp it. This depicts earth mastering water. The two-edged sword defeats the penetrating force of the spear. Here water extinguishes fire. The spear, in turn, subdues the hacking effect of the saber: Fire overcomes metal. The hacking action of saber, in its turn, can split the wooden staff; and so we see metal overcoming wood. Finally, the staff will break the bones of the open hand, and we see wood overcoming earth.

Each weapon is also paired with a tai chi movement. The open hand, for example, is paired with central balance, a term used to express the inner poise and assurance from which all other movements should proceed. Step and look left is related to metal and so is hard by nature. In action, a step and look to the left is followed by a right fist. If we study the cycle of construction, we find that metal is produced from earth and so, as a result of this association, the right fist should be delivered with inner poise and assurance.

Water depicts a special type of retreat. This is not the full flight of a defeated army but the tactical surrender of a useless position. In terms of the tai chi postures, it means to step back and it possesses the quality of suppleness. When the hardness of metal supports the pliability of water, we have a defensive position that is flexible. But it could become an offensive position in an instant. Look right is the movement related to wood, and it is said to embody might. When associated with water, the move implies a supple strength. Advance is associated with fire and refers to the offensive movement of stepping ahead. Coupled with wood, the natural ferocity of fire is fueled and increased. As you can see, the creative sequence is applied in an offensive manner.

The destructive sequence is applied in exactly the opposite manner, defensively. In this sequence, we see the phases, in the form of the elements, used to counteract each other. Earth overcomes water, and water subdues fire. Fire counters metal, which, in turn, subdues wood. The two cycles can also be understood in terms of expansion, represented by the aggressive pattern, and contraction, represented by the defensive pattern.

太極

Therapeutic Benefits of Tai Chi

Tai chi chuan is recognized as the most difficult of all the martial arts to use successfully in self-defense. This is primarily because of the problems in developing and applying the many internal energies such as chin. Even learning to understand these energies is a lengthy process. Fortunately, tai chi is an extremely interesting and enjoyable art to practice. And requirements for equipment and space are absolutely minimal: Tai chi can be practiced almost anywhere that a few square yards of space are available. Most importantly, its health benefits are readily apparent to practitioners from the very beginning of training.

Tai chi is a gentle art, so gentle that people of almost any age or physical condition can undertake it. In fact, many prominent teachers began their careers teaching tai chi late in life. Today, many different types of tai chi organizations have sprung up, each specializing in unique forms. Some of these groups have even designed instructional techniques specifically for older people, and private research centers now study the healing effects of tai chi.

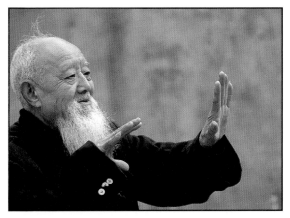

In the modern age, tai chi chuan's most significant contribution will probably not be considered its martial applications. Most likely, tai chi will be most valued for its contributions to good health. Recently, researchers have begun to conduct special studies not only on tai chi, but also on a number of traditional medical treatments including chi kung, acupuncture, and herbal remedies. The reason for this interest is clear: Many of these exercises and treatments are inex-

REDUCING FALL-RELATED INJURIES

One study, underwritten by the National Institute on Aging, reported that elderly tai chi practitioners demonstrated a 25 percent reduction in the number of falls they experienced. The study itself was conducted over a 12-year period by such notable medical institutions as the Centers for Disease Control and Prevention, Washington University School of Medicine, Emory University, Harvard, and Yale. The study concluded that balance training may work not simply because it improves balance itself, but because it increases awareness of personal limitations, enabling the practitioner to compensate.

Working in close connection with a tai chi master, the number of movements in the tai chi set was reduced from 108 to only 10 of the most important. For each group of participants, the study was conducted over a ten-week period. Even though the instructional period was brief, the benefits of the training typically lasted 1.5 years.

The results indicate that only 15 minutes of daily tai chi practice by the elderly could significantly reduce the number of fall-related injuries. At present, billions of medical dollars are spent annually caring for the elderly after injuries of this type. Couple this figure with the pain and inconvenience suffered by the victims, and one has a very good reason to promote tai chi.

pensive, easily accessible to the general public and, quite often, remarkably effective. Another reason is that researchers are trying to establish, in a definitive way, exactly which of the many claims of traditional medicine work and, if so, why they do.

Tai chi's fluid movements, always spiraling and bending, actually massage the internal organs, releasing them from damaging constrictions brought about by such factors as stress, poor posture, and difficult working conditions. This is one of the main health benefits of practicing tai chi. Some of the other purported benefits of regular tai chi practice that are currently under investigation include improved circulation, breathing, digestion, and flexion of limbs; stress management; relief from high blood pressure, back pain, and insomnia; and better overall health.

At this time, we do not have an abundance of clinical data describing the physical effects of tai chi. There are several reasons for this shortage of scientific data. Modern clinical research is really just beginning in this field. As we have already seen, it was not until the middle of this century that people knew anything at all about tai chi, even in China. In the Western world, the art has only gained popularity in the last two or three decades. Aside from the general level of interest, however, there is a cultural reason why more studies have not yet been conducted. In China, not everything has to be proven in a clinical study before it is accepted by the public. Since the effects of tai chi are obvious to those who practice it, this informal type of evidence has, generally speaking, proved satisfactory. The Chinese, then, have not had any particular reason to conduct clinical studies on the effects of tai chi.

Even from a rudimentary examination of the Western medical establishment, it is quite clear that its design pays little more than lip service to the idea of preventative care. Pharmaceutical companies, public and private hospitals, nursing homes, and many supporting industries depend on great numbers of people being sick. If more people were well, many of these corporations would simply disappear.

太極
Conclusion

In China a great deal of emphasis is placed on teaching people to keep themselves healthy. In fact, many Chinese tai chi masters have said that it is their obligation to teach tai chi for just this reason. These masters know that a strong country depends on a healthy population. So they teach tai chi because they believe this art will not only prevent disease but actually cure it efficiently and inexpensively.

More than 70 years ago, tai chi instructor Chen Wei-Ming said that tai chi strengthens the people and the country, but only if it retains its connection to the original principles. Otherwise, he says, tai chi will lose its essence and become more of a concern than a service.

In the middle of this century, another practitioner of equal renown, Cheng Man-ch'ing, eloquently expressed the same concern. There is good reason for calling tai chi chuan "the great ultimate," he said. Tai chi practitioners are able to neutralize hardness and speed, and they enjoy first place among martial artists. But that's not all. Tai chi chuan strengthens the weak, heals the sick, invigorates the debilitated, and encourages the timid. This, said Man-chi'ing, is truly the way to strengthen not just the individual, but the race, and the nation as well. The leaders who desire to ease the people's suffering cannot afford to overlook this.

A good practitioner is said to read only the best books, seek out the greatest teachers, and practice always with the instructions in mind. We can use intellectual knowledge of the art to direct and improve our practice. But this is only possible if we do indeed practice. Without practice, intellectual knowledge is essentially useless.

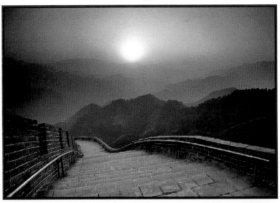

There is something else to remember, too: Tai chi is learned neither quickly nor without effort. While it can be practiced alone, it is learned only through instruction by others. And our instructors are indebted, as we are, to the efforts of those who have gone before. We can best express our appreciation to these past masters by remaining true to the fundamental principles they have demonstrated. When we are proficient in applying these abstract ideas to our daily practice, we will have received and understood the wisdom of the tai chi transmission.

INDEX

A

Aboriginal thought, 11–12

Achillea millefolium, 40

Acquired chi, 107

Acupoints

  chin and, 219–220

  names, meaning of, 177

  transcultural recognition of, 178

  understanding, 179–186

Acupressure, 189–190

Acupuncture

  acceptance of, 186–189

  as analgesia, 187

  channels, 166, 179–186, 219–220

  chi and, 99, 176

  effectiveness of, 187–189

  history of, 184–185

  theory behind, 175–176

  World Health Organization endorsement, 180

Advance movement, 228

Agility, in *The Five Character Secret*, 211

Aging

  chi kung and, 119, 140–141

  tai chi chuan and, 236

Alchemy, 88, 89

Anesthesia, chi kung as, 154–155

Animal behavior, chi kung and, 130–135

Art, Taoist, 75–80, 90–91. *See also* Calligraphy; Painting.

Artemisia vulgaris, 190

Auras, 130, 155–156

Auscultation and olfaction, 164

B

Back pain, 237

Baihui point, 139

Balance

  creation and, 52–53

C

D

E

H

I

U

UCLA Center for East-West Medicine, 188

Understanding, types of, 59

V

Vajrayana Buddhists, 128

Vedic literature, 114–115

Vitality, in *The Five Character Secret*, 213

W

Wang Chen-yeuh, 209

Ward off movement, 224

Water
  in five element theory, 168–174, 225–228
  five weapons and, 228–234

The Way, finding, 58–69.
  See also Tao.

Weaponry, tai chi, 228–234

Web of life, 173

Wei chi, 155–157

Weight underside, 108–111

Wen Wang, 35

White Clouded Temple, 201

WHO (World Health Organization), 180, 189

Wilhelm, Richard, 43–44

Wind chi, 113

Wisdom mind, 59–60

Wood
  in five element theory, 168–174, 225–228
  five weapons and, 228–234

World Health Organization (WHO), 180, 189

Wu chi, 50

Wu T'ang Temple, 201

Wu Yu-hsiang, 209, 210

Y

Yang. See Yin and yang.

Yang Ch'eng Fu, 208, 210

Yang Lu-ch'uan, 205–208